Breast-Feeding Today

Candace Woessner
Judith Lauwers
Barbara Bernard

Avery Publishing Group
Garden City Park, New York

Cover Design: William Gonzalez and Rudy Shur
Cover Photo: Catanzaro & Mahdessian Photography, Los Angeles, CA.
Original Illustrations: Vicki Rae Chelf and Pamela Tapia
In-House Editor: Joanne Abrams

Library of Congress Cataloging-in-Publication Data

Woessner, Candace, 1944-
Breastfeeding today: a mother's companion / Candace Woessner, Judith Lauwers, Barbara Bernard.—2nd ed.
p. cm.
Includes bibliographical references and index.
ISBN 0-89529-694-2
1. Breast feeding. I. Lauwers, Judith, 1949- . II. Bernard, Barbara, 1949- . III. Title.
RJ216.W718 1996
649.33—dc20 91-15434
CIP

Printed in the United States of America

10 9 8 7 6 5 4 3 2 1

Contents

This book is dedicated to
Walter, Dwight, and Kimberly Woessner
David, Christopher, and Michael Lauwers
and
Dan, Jennifer, Meghan, and Michael Bernard.

Without their love and patience,
it would never have become a reality.

Acknowledgments

We are grateful for the editorial contributions of Kathleen Auerbach, whose resolute attention to research and detail greatly aided us in our endeavor to present accurate, up-to-date information. Also deserving of special thanks are Vicki Rae Chelf and Pamela Tapia, whose artistry produced the unique drawings that appear throughout the book. Finally, we recognize the exceptional talents of Joanne Abrams, our editor, who persisted with patience and tenacity to cultivate our talents and extract a work of which we can be proud.

Foreword

My job here is to get everyone, male and female alike, so excited about breastfeeding that they will not even consider the alternative—cow's milk. We must remember that cow's milk was designed for a calf. No human has ever grown like a calf. That milk was assembled to feed that large animal with its proportionately small brain. Try to avoid it. There is plenty of time to drink it later on in life, if one finds it necessary to do so. (You should also remember when you drink it that you are stealing it from the calf.)

When I started my pediatric practice in the early 1950s, breastfeeding was looked upon as a peasant occupation. Modern women could disregard it because it was confining and not very scientific. The perception that seemed to be prominent then was of the barefoot woman, pregnant, nursing one child while two or three other children were tearing about destroying the mother's house, health, and sanity. No one wanted that image.

We doctor-types encouraged new mothers to take up the bottle because we wanted to be more in control of the intake. We knew that in order to thrive, a baby needed two ounces of some standard formula per pound per every twenty-four hours. How can you count the ounces if a woman is breastfeeding the baby? (Incidentally, much of the information provided to us was put together by the formula companies, who were anxious to please. I now think I know why they wanted to help us so much.)

It was frustrating to see the newborn baby's weight drop so much in those first few days. We told the mother struggling to establish nursing, "Why not give the poor, starving, little thing at least a few ounces of milk from the bottle while you are waiting for your milk to come in?" We made the new mother feel so guilty and anxious that her milk dried up even before it began to flow. What happens to the milk supply may be more a function of what's going on in the mother's head than what's going on in her breasts. We were not very supportive. We set her up for failure. But what did we know?

Now we know all the beautiful and wonderful things that can happen if a baby is breast-fed. Research has proven all these things; somehow we had been reluctant to accept the breasts as the obvious way to feed an infant. All the other mammals on earth have used them. Did we think that if we ignored them we would not suffer the wrath of Mother Nature?

When I started practice, I counted about one child in ten who needed to be changed from cow's milk to soy or goat's milk or to a meat-based milk substitute. The symptoms varied from colic to rashes to vomiting and diarrhea. My recent analysis of the newborns in my practice revealed an allergy to milk incidence of about one in two. I also stumbled onto the connection between cow's milk intolerance and the rather high incidence of ear infections and streptococcal sore throat. It bothers me now to hear of a child who seems to be happy with breast milk, but is sick nonetheless. In most of these cases, it is the dairy products the mother is eating and drinking that contribute to this sensitivity. Some of that cow's milk protein goes right through to the mother's breast milk and irritates the poor innocent thing. It somehow lowers the child's resistance, and the viruses and germs that are always around invade this susceptible host. In the absence of irritants such as this, breast-fed babies seem to have a *higher* resistance to infection than do formula-fed babies.

The authors of this book have used a common-sense approach to breastfeeding. Now that we all know that it is important in feeding infants, it is time to get the milk flowing. The problem might be that the grandmothers that I counseled are still around and might be saying, "We used the bottle, dearie, and it was easy. Even got your father in on the feedings."

But try not to be dissuaded by those who think that the bottle is the easy way out. It is not right for our children. Nurse, nurse, nurse. Even after a stressful delivery or a Cesarean, you will be able to nurse the baby. Many women have adopted babies and successfully nursed them. When a baby sucks on the breast, a message goes up to the brain: "You won't believe this, brain, but there is a baby out there." The brain sends the appropriate hormones out to the breasts, and the milk flows. It takes a little doing, but it can work.

It would be ideal to have the authors of this book in your neighborhood to give aid and support to your efforts. Most lactation experts know that 90 to 95 percent of women are able to nurse, given a few instructions and some encouragement. Unfortunately, the authors cannot be right there in the room with you. You may have to enlist your own team. Your husband and relatives may be helpful, but sometimes they won't know what to do or say, except, "Give him a bottle!"

This book gives accurate information about a subject that has long been an art form. Practical tips about nursing are based on scientific knowledge of hormones, the anatomy of the baby's mouth, the anatomy of the milk ducts, and the way in which they all interact.

Traditionally, when lay people write books about something that appears to invade the territory of a professional, the writers often end a technical passage or a discussion of a new therapeutic idea with, "Please, call your doctor." I am that doctor, and I get those calls all the time. Doctors like easy ones like, "If I break a leg, should I have it put in a cast?" But when mothers call and say, "I don't think the baby is getting enough milk from nursing," we usually give the routine, "Better switch to the bottle, Ma'am." What a cop-out. What do we know? But books like this are helping us learn.

For a number of years, we relied on mothers who had nursed their babies and subsequently formed support groups for new mothers. They had learned through personal experience, and were very helpful. It now seems that a new professional group of lactation consultants is growing and achieving great success because of their advanced training in this important field. Lactation consultants can combine the science and the emotional support. It would be worth seeking one of these experts out even before the baby is born.

A well-documented study published in our *Pediatrics* journal two years ago followed the progress of several completely breast-fed babies over the first eighteen months of life. None of them had eaten any baby food. None had been sick. Allergies were minimal. They were not anemic, and were cheerful, healthy, and had gained well. The mothers, of course, were healthy and well-nourished.

Nevertheless, nursing mothers still have questions and problems. Some of the most frequently reported problems are inadequate weight gain, colic, and fussiness.

I have found out that many problems of nursing babies are due to a bad positioning of the baby at the breast. This is also one of the most common causes of sore nipples.

Food sensitivities are another cause of infant problems. In fact, I believe that they are one of the chief factors in the triggering of colic, sickness, and allergy symptoms, and that milk is the first food on the list of offenders. Soy, corn, wheat, eggs, and the rest of the common "good, healthy" foods follow apace. Rotating the diet is the best way to avoid these sensitivities; try not to eat the same food every day.

The obstetrician might take some of the blame for the high incidence of allergies. He or she usually urges the pregnant woman to chug down a quart of milk a day so that baby's calcium needs will be realized. In some cases, this will make the baby sensitive to dairy products even before birth. Other sources of calcium could be considered.

The pediatrician, also, has been responsible for the appearance of many food sensitivities. We were taught to start the solids in the first few weeks because it "would help the baby sleep through the night sooner." Wrong. All we did was to make these infants allergic to these foods, and many of them did not outgrow those allergies. Their intestinal tract was not meant to digest anything other than mother's milk. So now we have the parents wait until the infant is over six months, or until the teeth start to come in at eight to ten months or the child is grabbing food off the parents' plates.

Another possible cause of problems in nursing infants is the overuse of the pacifier. I have seen a few babies who seemed completely happy for weeks, but had gained nothing. The mother admitted that whenever her baby's mouth was open, she stuck the pacifier into it. Most babies let the world know when their stomachs are empty, but for some it is no big deal. These unaware mothers should have been putting the babies on their breasts every two hours or so.

When trying to settle my own children down after a feeding, bottle or breast, I would thump on the upper abdomen as if I were testing a melon for ripeness. If "ready," I would sit the child upright and gently rock him or her back and forth, left and right, until the bubble found the opening to the esophagus. I would be rewarded with a dry burp.

When a baby refuses to nurse and has a runny nose, it might be due to an ear infection. Sucking creates a vacuum in the nasopharynx and empties the air from the Eustachian tube; this tugs at the inflamed eardrum, usually causing the baby to scream. Have the doctor check for an ear infection.

When your family and friends want you to quit nursing the baby at one or two or even three years of age and you don't want to, tell them that your doctor says that you have to keep it up. (Dr. Smith, that is.)

I am delighted with this book—by the way it is organized and the encouragement it offers to the woman (and her family) who wants to nurse because she knows it is the best thing for her and her baby. I like the summary panels scattered throughout the book to give a quick overview of the text.

The new mother is proud of her ability to nurse, but society is not quite ready for her to nurse fully exposed in public. A woman was nursing her infant in a mall in a large city a couple of years ago. A local merchant felt she was hurting his business and came out of his store and told her so, even though she was discreetly covering her chest and her baby. The next Saturday she gathered a few of her nursing mother friends and they sat on benches facing his store and had a giant suck-in. Hooray for women's lib and this great book.

Lendon H. Smith, M.D.
Portland, Oregon

Preface

Today's woman. Who is she? What is the profile of a mother today? She is the meal planner, house cleaner, launderer, and nursemaid. She is the family financial planner, homemaker, and chauffeur. She is the woman who volunteers her time in the school, the church, the hospital, and community organizations.

She is also the college-educated woman who chose to remain at home with her children rather than pursue a career. She is the career woman who postponed starting a family until she was firmly established in her profession. She is the single mother struggling to earn a living for her family, or the adolescent living at home with her parents and raising a baby. She is the ethnic woman, continents away from her homeland and family, raising her children in a strange land. She is the young mother working toward finishing her college degree. She is the mother whose income from a full- or part-time job is needed to help her family keep up with inflation, or the woman who must turn to food assistance programs to ensure her family's well-being.

No one profile can adequately describe today's woman. And yet, with such diverse backgrounds and interests, women today share one common challenge. Many are attempting to breastfeed in a society that is still emerging from an era in which babies were almost universally formula-fed. Because their own mothers frequently lack experience with breastfeeding, women today are turning to parent groups, books, and self-education for assistance and support.

This book addresses you—today's woman—and your diverse

needs. It acknowledges one other special quality of today's woman: she expects to be treated as an equal partner in the physician-patient relationship. She is an informed consumer who questions and persists until she is satisfied. Today's woman works as part of a team with her doctor and other health care providers, questioning and seeking the information necessary for making her own decisions about her health and that of her family.

The purpose of this book is to offer advice and support to breastfeeding women. Mothers who are breastfeeding for the first time, as well as those with previous nursing experience, will benefit from the warm and supportive manner in which topics are discussed. If this book were to have only one purpose, it would be to reassure you that most of what you will experience while breastfeeding is normal, and that your emotions and concerns are shared by many others. You will manage breastfeeding and parenting in your own way, adapting it to your lifestyle and personal goals.

The text is organized in a manner that, we feel, will make the information most accessible. Chapter 1 is presented in a question-and-answer style in order to raise the issues that confront women as they consider the option of breastfeeding. Topics presented in this chapter are discussed in detail throughout the remainder of the book. Because you should ideally be learning about breastfeeding during pregnancy, Chapter 2 discusses issues that the pregnant woman should consider at this time. Next, you will need basic information about breastfeeding management before actually beginning to nurse your baby. Chapter 3 discusses the anatomy and physiology of the breast, explaining how the breast makes milk and how the milk becomes available for the baby. Chapter 4 treats the topic of breast milk, advising you of its special properties and of ways to preserve its quality. During both pregnancy and lactation, sound nutrition is important; this is the theme of Chapter 5.

Once you have a clear understanding of these principles, you will be ready to begin breastfeeding. Chapter 6 will guide you through the early days, as you and your baby become accustomed to each other and learn how to manage the initial feedings. Situations that may interfere with breastfeeding success are discussed in Chapter 7, with descriptions of both the problems and the measures to correct them. Physical adjustments related to a mother's postpartum recovery are presented in Chapter 8, with emphasis on the need for rest following delivery. Chapter 9 will acquaint you with normal behaviors of a newborn, including patterns of early feedings and weight gain. The many social adjustments that confront the breastfeeding family are addressed in Chapter 10, with advice on how to deal with unsupportive people and suggestions for helping family members accommodate themselves to breastfeeding.

After getting off to a good start, you may confront obstacles in the early weeks and months that, if not understood, can result in untimely weaning. Chapter 11 will help you to fit breastfeeding into your life, and will educate you about those aspects of breastfeeding that are related to your child's early growth and behavior. The discussion of the baby's growth and development is continued in Chapter 12, with a focus on events that occur in the later months of breastfeeding. As you move toward the end of the breastfeeding experience, you will need advice about making the transition to other forms of nourishment. This information is presented in Chapter 12.

The final three chapters deal with specific issues that do not confront every nursing mother. Since so many women today are interested in breastfeeding after their return to work, this topic is treated in depth in Chapter 13, with many helpful hints for the working mother. Special birth and health situations that may affect breastfeeding are discussed in Chapter 14, with practical advice for managing nursings. Finally, special breastfeeding aids and devices are described in Chapter 15, with instructions for proper use.

Following each chapter, we have supplied a summary of essential points that were discussed. These summaries are intended as ready reference tools. We anticipate that you will wish to review specific information at each stage of breastfeeding. By turning to the "At A Glance" section, you will be able to locate this information without rereading an entire chapter.

It is our hope that the tone of the book will offer comfort and understanding as you learn more about nurturing your baby. Ideally, a breastfeeding mother has access to a supportive lay counselor, a lactation consultant, or another type of breastfeeding helper. We have attempted to transcend the impersonality of the printed page and approach you in the manner of a counselor who, over time, would develop a warm relationship with you, offer advice and support, and promote feelings of self-confidence and self-reliance.

Although your baby is just as likely to be a girl as a boy, our language, unfortunately, has not provided us with a genderless pronoun. Therefore, to avoid using the awkward "he/she" or the impersonal "it" when referring to the baby, the masculine pronouns "he," "him," and "his" have been used throughout this book. Similarly, we have used the masculine pronouns to refer to doctors and the feminine pronouns to refer to nurses and other health care providers, without meaning to imply that this is in any way the preferred situation. These decisions have been made in the interest of simplicity and clarity.

1

Questions Mothers Ask

Breastfeeding is rapidly regaining popularity as a way of feeding the newborn. Although formula feeding is still common, the medical community and general public are gradually becoming aware of the benefits of breastfeeding. However, misconceptions about breastfeeding and a lack of accurate information on the subject may have left you feeling confused and uncertain about infant feeding options. To help you make a decision with which you will feel comfortable, this chapter answers the most commonly asked questions regarding breastfeeding. Specific information and step-by-step instructions on key topics are presented in later chapters.

Why is breastfeeding better for my baby than formula feeding?

Breast milk is uniquely designed to promote optimum health and growth in the human infant. It is more easily digested and efficiently utilized by the baby than is any other form of nourishment. Breast milk is a living, changing food; it contains enzymes and living cells that cannot be manufactured in a laboratory. These factors help to prevent or delay allergies, protect the infant from infectious diseases, and reduce the occurrence of respiratory and digestive infections. The specific make-up of the milk varies to suit the changing needs of the baby as he grows. In addition, breastfeeding promotes healthy oral development, satisfies sucking needs, and enhances bonding and skin-to-skin contact between mother and child. See Chapter 4 for more information on the value of breast milk.

How can breast milk protect my baby from disease?

Because you have already been exposed to a number of different diseases, your body has developed immunities to them. You will pass these immunities on to your baby through your breast milk. Also, breast milk contains elements that will line your baby's digestive system and protect it from attack by certain organisms. Other elements in your milk will either destroy bacteria or retard its growth, thus protecting your baby in still another way. Neither formula nor pasteurized cow's milk has these protective properties. Even the milk from other mothers will not be identical to your own breast milk, which is suited to meet the special needs of your baby. For more information on the value of breast milk, see Chapter 4.

What advantages will there be for me?

With the beginning of breastfeeding, a special closeness will develop between you and your baby that will continue throughout your life together. You may have a sense of self-fulfillment as a result of doing something that no one else can do for your baby. In addition, breastfeeding is economical and convenient. While your own nutritional intake may have to increase, the cost of additional food for you will be less than the expense of bottles and formula. By breastfeeding, you will also avoid the time-consuming and frustrating task of preparing sterilized bottles of formula while listening to your baby's hunger cries. Your breast milk will be constantly available, sterile, and at the proper temperature. Since you will not need to prepare or transport bottles, travel and other outside activities will be more convenient. And, during feedings, you will have a free hand for such enjoyable activities as reading and cuddling older children.

There are also physical advantages for you as a breastfeeding mother. Your baby's suckling will stimulate your uterus to return to its prepregant size sooner, and thus reduce the chances of postpartum complications. The increased caloric demand that nursing will place on your body may make it easier for you to control your weight after delivery Also, because you will be able to rest during feedings, night feedings will be less demanding and can even take place in bed. As an added bonus, the stools and spit-up of a breast-fed baby are less offensive than those of a bottle-fed infant and do not stain, making baby care more pleasant.

Aren't there some drawbacks to breastfeeding?

The most common problems usually occur during the early weeks of breastfeeding. Most of these are temporary, and with time and proper breastfeeding management can be avoided or alleviated. Uncomfortable breast fullness often occurs during the first few days after the baby's birth, but subsides after about ten days. Early, frequent feedings usually prevent this from becoming a problem. Although initial nipple soreness may occur, it is temporary and can be avoided or relieved by using the techniques that are discussed in Chapter 7. Some mothers initially produce excess milk that leaks from the breasts. Such leaking usually subsides by four to six weeks postpartum. During the transitional period, nursing pads or breast shells can be used to control leakage.

As your baby's only source of nutrition, you will have to be available for feedings, and a breast-fed baby needs to be fed more frequently than a formula-fed baby. While this may seem to restrict your time, feeding methods really have very little effect on time spent with a young baby. Babies thrive on closeness and attention, especially in the early weeks. During the first six weeks or so, plan on taking your baby with you on most occasions. As your baby grows, the intervals between feedings will increase, and he will begin to become interested in the world around him. Then he will more readily accept care from others, allowing you more time for outside activities as he matures. Your initial investment of time spent with your baby will provide him with the security he needs to develop self-confidence.

How will I know if my baby is getting enough breast milk?

You will know that your baby is getting enough to eat if he looks healthy, has good skin tone, and grows at a normal rate. Also, if your child has six to ten wet diapers a day (or three to five super-absorbent disposable diapers) without producing dark concentrated urine and without taking any supplements or water, you will know that he is being well-nourished by your breast milk.

By observing your baby and taking cues from him, you will learn to manage feedings to satisfy his needs. Nurse him when he begins to stir, before fussing develops into crying. Space feedings no more than three hours apart during the day, and as long as he likes at night. Observe how he sucks while nursing—quickly at the beginning of the feeding, more slowly as milk is released into his mouth, and then quickly again as the amount of milk decreases.

What medical conditions might prevent me from breastfeeding?

With proper information, good nursing techniques, and adequate emotional support, more than 95 percent of all women can nurse successfully. There are, however, some medical situations that prohibit safe breastfeeding. These conditions include some forms of long-term drug therapy, unstable diabetes, congestive heart failure, eclampsia, typhoid, some types of breast reduction surgery, and long-term insufficient nutrition. Normally, a woman with active tuberculosis should not breastfeed until treatment has been administered for at least one week and she is no longer infectious; both mother and baby must be treated in this case. Since not enough is known about Acquired Immune Deficiency Syndrome (AIDS), the consequences for an infant who is breastfed by an AIDS mother are not clear. Therefore, until more research has been performed, breastfeeding is not recommended.

Most medical conditions are compatible with breastfeeding. The health profession is continuing to learn more about the special needs of these mothers and babies. In addition, support groups are often available to provide both practical advice and emotional support.

Can a nervous person breastfeed?

Even if you are an anxious person, you can breastfeed successfully. The hormones involved in the production and flow of breast milk have a relaxing effect on the body. This may help to decrease your feelings of anxiety. Extreme tension sometimes blocks the release of milk. This release, called the letdown reflex or milk ejection reflex, can be conditioned by setting up a routine for each feeding. Once the reflex has been conditioned, even intense anxiety seldom inhibits it. Specific suggestions for conditioning the letdown reflex are provided in Chapter 6.

Are there any women who simply cannot produce enough milk?

Years ago, many women were told that they were not producing an adequate amount of milk, or that their milk was drying up. Today, however, we know that they probably were not nursing frequently enough. More milk is produced each time the baby nurses, so to ensure a good milk supply, the most important thing you can do is to nurse often.

Only a very few women are unable to provide their baby's total nourishment due to insufficient milk-producing glands. There is no evidence that the inability to breastfeed is hereditary. However, certain types of breast surgery may interfere with the functional tissue of the breast. If you have had breast surgery, be sure to check with your surgeon to find out if the milk-producing tissue was involved and, if so, to what degree it was affected.

Will the size or shape of my breasts affect my ability to nurse?

The appearance of your breasts has no bearing on your ability to produce sufficient milk. Size and shape are determined primarily by the outer, fatty layer of tissue. The milk-producing or functional tissue lies deep within the breast, and adds little to the size of the nonpregnant breast. It is the development of this unseen portion of the breast during pregnancy that affects milk production.

Will breastfeeding make my breasts sag?

Breastfeeding alone will not cause your breasts to sag. Pregnancy, increased breast size, lack of muscle tone, and hereditary factors are the primary causes of decreased firmness. Sagging, which sometimes results from changes that occur during pregnancy, is as common in women who choose to bottle feed as it is in breastfeeding women. While there is no clear evidence that sagging is directly related to breastfeeding, it is possible that the tissues may stretch when the lactating breast is very full of milk and the fluids that contribute to milk production. In breastfeeding women, increased breast size is most common during the first ten days after birth. After that time, the breast tissues usually return to their previous size, unless feedings are missed and the breasts become overly full. As a precautionary measure, therefore, it is a good idea to wear a support bra in order to prevent an excessive stretching of the tissues whenever the breasts are enlarged— during pregnancy, throughout the first ten days of lactation, and when the breasts are unusually full of milk. Women with large breasts may need to rely on a support bra at all times to prevent sagging, whether or not they choose to breastfeed.

What if I try breastfeeding and fail?

You may find breastfeeding difficult during the first few weeks, when you and your baby are still getting used to each other. As you both learn more about breastfeeding and begin to work as a team, breastfeeding will become more enjoyable and rewarding. Your extra efforts in the beginning will pay off in the development of a healthy, happy baby and a close mother-infant relationship. In addition, should you decide at any time that breastfeeding is not for you, you can easily switch to bottle feeding. If a baby is bottle-fed from birth, however, it takes a great effort to initiate breastfeeding beyond the first few weeks after birth.

Will breastfeeding make excessive demands on my body?

Breastfeeding will make demands on your body, but by eating

well and planning for adequate rest, you will be able to maintain your energy level and enthusiasm. One of the best ways to avoid fatige is to be sure to eat a quarter of your daily protein requirements (ten to fifteen grams) at breakfast. Rest whenever possible, and take a nap when your baby naps. Also, avoid too much physical activity during the early weeks, building up gradually to your prepregnant level by two to three months postpartum.

How can I be sure that my milk will be rich enough?

Unless your diet is extremely poor, the composition of your breast milk will be just as rich as any other woman's milk. Your baby will receive sufficient calories if he nurses long enough to take in the milk with high fat content that is present as he ends his nursing on a breast. To stimulate milk production, nurse every two to three hours. In addition, be certain to eat a well-balanced diet. This should ensure your baby's well-being and your own good health.

Several factors might mistakenly cause a woman to believe that her milk is not rich enough. The normal appearance of human milk is thin and watery compared with cow's milk, causing new mothers to think that it is nutritionally deficient. On the contrary, human milk is ideally suited to the growth rate of the human infant. In addition, the breast-fed baby nurses more often than the bottle-fed baby, because breast milk is digested more quickly. If a mother is unaware of the need to feed her baby frequently, she may believe that her milk is of poor quality. An infant's failure to gain weight may also incorrectly cause a woman to believe that her milk is not rich enough when, in fact, she is simply not nursing often enough. You can avoid these problems by nursing your baby whenever he is hungry.

Will I need to change my eating habits in order to breastfeed?

A nutritious diet is important for breastfeeding women, but establishing a proper diet need not be difficult. You will require roughly the same amount of nutrients while nursing that you needed during pregnancy. A good rule to follow is to eat three well-balanced meals and two nutritious snacks every day. Select foods from the four basic food groups, and distribute them evenly throughout the day. You will know that you are eating well if you feel good, look good, have enough energy to get through the day, and are resistant to common diseases such as colds and the flu.

What foods should I avoid?

There are no foods that must be strictly avoided while breastfeeding. However, you may find that certain foods bother your baby. Usually, these are foods that tend to cause gas. In addition, some babies exhibit allergic reactions to a few foods that are eaten by their mothers. Most commonly, these include milk, eggs, peanuts, and citrus fruits. Large amounts of caffeine may cause wakefulness in your baby, so limit the amount of coffee, tea, cola, and chocolate you consume if your baby seems to be overstimulated. The best advice is to eat all foods in moderation. Watch for signs of discomfort in your baby, and eliminate any foods that seem to cause problems. Most mothers are able to breastfeed their babies and still eat the foods they enjoy.

Is it possible for my baby to be allergic to my breast milk?

Babies sometimes have allergic reactions to something their mothers have eaten. Molecules from food can pass from the mother's stomach into her blood stream, and from there into her breast milk. If you are able to identify the offending food and eliminate it from your diet, your breastfeeding will not be affected. Your breast milk is perfectly suited to your baby and will pose no problems if you choose your foods wisely.

Will I ever be able to leave my baby with a sitter?

The typical woman today is involved in many activities outside the home. Breastfeeding need not keep you from taking part in these activities. Sometimes, you will be able to take your baby with you. At other times, you will be able to participate in your outside pursuits by leaving a relief bottle for your baby. Use either a breast pump or hand expression to relieve fullness and to collect breast milk that can be given to your baby when you are away. A cylindrical pump is ideally suited for this purpose. If you choose to prepare formula for relief bottles, be sure to empty your breasts by pumping or hand expression whenever feedings are missed.

By occasionally giving your baby a bottle, you will help to ensure his acceptance of an alternative feeding method. However, avoid introducing relief bottles until after your milk supply has been well-established. As a rule of thumb, the first bottle should be offered no earlier than six weeks postpartum, but no later than three months. See Chapter 11 for advice on the use of relief bottles.

Can I nurse in public without drawing attention to myself?

Nursing in public can be done comfortably and discreetly with amazing ease. If you remain relaxed and take a few common-sense precautions, most people will be unaware that you are nursing your baby. Before you attempt nursing in public, observe how other women nurse their babies discreetly, and then practice at home in front of a mirror or another person. You can nurse comfortably in public by giving careful attention to clothing and selecting an appropriate place for nursings. Time feedings so that your baby does not become so hungry that he cries and draws attention to himself. See Chapter 11 for more suggestions on how to nurse discreetly in public.

Can I breastfeed if I am going back to work?

A high percentage of new mothers today return to work a month or two after their babies are born. It is taxing to be both a mother and a working woman, whether breastfeeding or not, and the decision to breastfeed and maintain a full-time job is not an easy one to make. However, many women find that they can successfully combine these two activities, and that continuing to breastfeed often makes the return to work easier. It does require careful planning and organization. Specific suggestions are presented in Chapter 13.

If I have a Cesarean birth, will I still be able to nurse my baby?

The way in which your baby is born will not affect your ability to breastfeed. The hormones essential for breastfeeding are triggered by the delivery of the placenta, even when the placenta is delivered surgically. You may have a slower start because of your baby's drowsiness or your delayed recovery from the anesthetic. In addition, you will require more rest because you have had major surgery, and may need to find ways to position your baby so that he does not irritate your incision. These problems are temporary, however, and will not impair your long-term breastfeeding success. Further discussions of breastfeeding by Cesarean mothers appear in Chapter 14.

If my baby is born prematurely, will I be able to breastfeed?

In the case of premature birth, breastfeeding will be delayed, but in time it may be possible for you to nurse successfully. After delivery, you should begin pumping as soon as possible to build your milk supply. Breast milk from the mother of a premature baby has higher concentrations of nutrients that are specially suited to the baby's needs,[1] and your doctor may request that you provide your baby with this milk during the early days. Your milk will first be given to your baby by tube, then by bottle, and finally by breast. Much of the success of breastfeeding a premature baby depends on his birth weight and the development of his sucking reflex. See Chapter 14 for additional information on nursing a premature baby.

Can a mother produce enough milk to breastfeed twins?

Your body can make as much milk as your babies need. You will have to rest, maintain a good diet, minimize stress, and make sure that your breasts are stimulated by adequate suckling. If the babies seem hungry all of the time, nurse more often, and your body will make more milk. By planning a nursing schedule and evaluating your priorities, you will be able to nurse twins, or even triplets, successfully. For specific suggestions, see Chapter 14.

Is it safe to nurse during pregnancy?

Unless feedings cause frequent contractions, you will be able to safely nurse during pregnancy. If you do experience contractions, it is advisable to wean your toddler to prevent premature labor. You will need more rest and vitamin-rich foods if you continue nursing during pregnancy. Because of the changes in the composition of your milk, your toddler may initiate weaning as your delivery date approaches. If you decide to wean, see Chapter 12 for ways to wean your toddler gradually and with a minimum of emotional stress.

If I decide not to breastfeed but find that my baby is allergic to formula, will I be able to switch to breastfeeding?

It takes a lot of determination to get a late start with breastfeeding, but with perseverance you can be successful, especially if you have delivered recently. Set aside several weeks to concentrate solely on breastfeeding, encouraging your baby to nurse as often as possible so that your milk supply is steadily increased.

What problems will I have as a single parent?

Because of the demands on your time, breastfeeding your baby will require extra determination. Since you may be working full-time and have sole responsibility for the care of your home and family, you should carefully evaluate your priorities. Eliminate inessential tasks and find short cuts for others. Develop relationships with other single breastfeeding mothers for mutual support and the trading of favors. Chapter 13 offers further suggestions that will help you to fit breastfeeding into your work schedule.

AT A GLANCE

Questions Mothers Ask

The Pros and Cons of Breastfeeding

- Breast milk provides the infant with special nutrients that cannot be obtained from formula.
- Advantages for the breastfeeding mother include a sense of self fulfillment; physical benefits, such as ease in controlling weight; the avoidance of bottle-feeding-related expenses; and the convenience of preparation-free feedings.
- Drawbacks include early temporary discomforts and the need for the mother to be available for feedings.

Ensuring Breastfeeding Success

- 95% of all women have the potential to breastfeed successfully.
- All types of women—nervous or calm, active or sedentary—can nurse successfully.
- Frequent feedings of sufficient duration will ensure that your baby gets plenty of nourishment.
- A mother whose diet is well-balanced can breastfeed successfully and without great expense.
- Eat all foods in moderation, eliminating only those that cause discomfort in you or your baby.

Adapting Breastfeeding Techniques to Different Situations

- Most breast-fed babies can occasionally be fed with a bottle of breast milk or formula, enabling the mother to pursue activities outside the home.
- With practice, the breastfeeding mother can discreetly nurse in public.
- The mother who had a Cesarean birth can breastfeed successfully.
- Special situations such as working, having twins, and premature birth do not necessarily prevent breastfeeding.

2

Planning for Baby's Arrival

Breastfeeding will get your child off to the best possible nutritional start. In order to help breastfeeding go smoothly—especially during the first few weeks, when you will be adjusting to life with a new baby—take time now to plan and prepare for breastfeeding. A good diet, plenty of rest, and proper exercise will get you in shape for labor and delivery, in addition to providing the energy stores needed for nursing. Educating yourself through the information in this book and preparing your breasts for nursing will help you to master the necessary mechanics. Planning where in your home you will nurse, considering which clothing will be suitable for breastfeeding, and arranging for friends and relatives to help out during the first few weeks will allow you to relax and concentrate on the care of your new baby.

Breastfeeding is most successful when those around you—your relatives, friends, and health care providers—are supportive of your efforts. Share your enthusiasm and breastfeeding knowledge with them and let them know that their support is very important to you. It will also help if the medical team you choose is willing to answer your questions about breastfeeding and to assist you in your efforts to have close contact with your baby at all times.

CHOOSING SUPPORTIVE HEALTH CARE

By the time you begin to seriously consider infant feeding options, you will probably have already chosen the health care provider who will attend you during pregnancy and birth.

However, other aspects of health care should also be considered as you plan for your baby's arrival. Both the hospital in which you and your baby will spend your first hours together and the doctor who will provide your child with his first medical care should be selected with an eye to maximizing breastfeeding success. By carefully examining your options and choosing those that are most compatible with your philosophies of infant care, you will be laying a firm foundation for a satisfactory breastfeeding relationship.

Choosing Hospital and Birthing Center Care

Your doctor will be able to attend your baby's birth only at a facility in which he has been granted privileges to practice. During your pregnancy, you should explore the health care options open to you for childbirth and your hospital stay. Policies that allow contact between you, your baby, and your baby's father will be most conducive to breastfeeding success. To increase awareness and eye contact during delivery, it is preferable to avoid the use of drugs that might make you or your baby drowsy. Ask that the administration of eye drops used to prevent infection be delayed so that your baby will be able to see you clearly during your first minutes together. If you are permitted to hold and nurse your baby soon after birth, your relationship will get off to a good start.

Consider policies that will affect your early days of breastfeeding. When the second nursing takes place within four hours of the first, and when there are at least nine nursings during each twenty-four hour period, breastfeeding is most successful. A sound breastfeeding routine will be most quickly established if you can arrange to have your baby with you in your room, so that he can nurse whenever he is hungry. Your center may offer several types of **rooming-in** arrangements. Some allow your baby to go back to the nursery—either when you wish to rest or at regularly scheduled times. Some facilities restrict visitors or limit rooming-in to nonvisiting hours. Other centers keep the babies in the nursery but bring them to their mothers for **demand** or **need feedings** (feedings that take place when the baby indicates a need to be fed). If you are able to make use of a hospital birthing room, you will probably be able to have your baby with you at all times. In birth centers, mothers, babies, and fathers are usually kept together for the entire stay (twelve to twenty-four hours).

Check with your own doctor and your baby's doctor to learn about the options that are open to you. If you are dissatisfied with your options, you may wish to consider changing doctors in order to utilize a facility that is more compatible with your needs. If your baby's doctor is sympathetic to your wishes, however, you may be able to make arrangements for special privileges such as round-the-clock need feedings. Be sure that your own physician is notified in writing of all such arrangements, and that once you are in your room, specific instructions are recorded on your medical chart. To prepare for your hospital stay, you may wish to explore the following policies and practices:

Insurance Coverage

- Is this hospital covered by your present insurance policy? If so, what percentage of the costs will be reimbursed?

Rooming-In

- What arrangements are available?
- What are the rooming-in hours?
- Is a specific type of room required (private or semiprivate)?
- What are the limitations, if any, when you have a roommate?
- Must you specify rooming-in prior to admission, or can you elect it during your stay?

Feeding Schedules

- What is the standard feeding schedule?
- What arrangements must be made for need feedings?
- How are nighttime feedings handled?

The First Nursing

- Where does the first nursing take place—in the delivery room or the recovery room?
- Can eye drops be delayed until after the first nursing?
- What time is allowed for the mother and father to interact with their baby after birth?

Drugs Used During Labor and Delivery

- What drugs are normally used during labor and delivery?
- What effect will specific drugs have on the responsiveness of mother and baby?

Visiting Privileges

- Who is allowed in the mother's room—father, grandparents, siblings, other relatives, friends?
- What are the visiting hours?
- Who is allowed in the room when the baby is present?
- Are there special visiting hours for fathers?
- Can the mother visit with other children in her room or in another portion of the hospital? Can the baby be present during these visits?

Selecting Your Baby's Doctor

In the excitement of getting things ready for your baby's arrival, do not overlook the important task of selecting pediatric care. Because your child will need to be under medical supervision for many years, you should thoroughly investigate all available services. Although the majority of infants are under the care of a physician, other options are available. A certified nurse-midwife is qualified to care for you and your baby. She is a registered nurse who has received special training in prenatal care, labor and delivery, and well-baby care. Well-baby care includes routine checkups to monitor growth and development and to administer regular inoculations. Nurse practitioners and nurse clinicians can also provide the care you need. They are registered nurses who have been trained to provide health services under the supervision of a physician. Consider the types of services you prefer and investigate those that are available in your area. This will help you choose a health care team whose philosophies will be compatible with your own and whose facilities will serve you well as your family grows.

It is wise to select medical care for your baby through recommendations from friends, relatives, your personal physician, or your clinic. Try to explore at least two or three different care providers. Look for one whose practice includes many breast-fed babies, who has calling times that enable you to reach him personally, and with whom you feel you can work well.

Before arranging for a consultation with a doctor, you may wish to investigate his background and hospital affiliation. Medical directories, which are available in most local libraries, provide information regarding the educational backgrounds and the hospital and society affiliations of physicians. Your county medical society too, can provide this information, and can also identify new physicians who may be eager to accommodate the needs of a new patient. For personal consumer recommendations on specific doctors throughout the United States, you can write to The People's Medical Society, 14 East Minor Street, Emmaus, PA 18049.

When you are satisfied with a doctor's medical standing, you should arrange for an office visit as early in your pregnancy as possible, preferably in the first trimester. During your visit, keep in mind that the manner in which a doctor answers your questions—his tone of voice, expression, and willingness to go into detail—may reveal more about his attitude than the answers themselves. Some issues you may wish to consider are:

Insurance Coverage

- Are the services of this doctor covered by your insurance policy? If so, what percentage of the costs will be reimbursed?

Availability

- How convenient is the doctor's office location?
- With which hospitals is the doctor affiliated? How close are they to your home and to your and your husband's places of business?
- What are the doctor's office hours? Is he available in the evenings and on weekends, as well as during the day?
- What times can the doctor be reached directly by phone?
- Does he have special call hours before or after regular office hours?

- Does the doctor practice independently, or with a group of other doctors? If with a group, would you be seen by one doctor, or by the group members on a rotating basis? What are the philosophies of the other group members? Can arrangements be made to see one particular doctor for all visits?
- How are emergency calls handled after regular office hours?
- If the doctor has an independent practice, who covers for him when he is not available? Is the covering doctor someone whose philosophies are compatible with yours?

Helpfulness

- Does the doctor seem willing to listen to your concerns and consider your point of view?
- Is he willing to take time with you and give you personal attention?
- Does he encourage parents to participate in decision making, especially concerning nonmedical issues such as sleeping arrangements, child care, and styles of parenting?
- How willing is he to discuss problems over the phone, in lieu of an office visit?

Care of the Breast-Fed Baby

- What are the doctor's recommendations on rooming-in?
- How long is he willing to delay treatment of your newborn's eyes, allowing you and your child time to bond?
- What are his recommendations for the time and location of the first nursing?
- Does he encourage frequent nursings both in the hospital and at home?
- In the hospital, what are his standing orders, i.e., his permanent instructions for the staff on the management of baby care and breastfeeding?
- How does his prescribed treatment of jaundice accommodate breastfeeding?
- What are his policies on vitamin, iron, and fluoride supplements?
- What is his schedule for routine checkups?

- What range of weight gain does he consider normal for breast-fed babies?
- What are his recommendations regarding the use of supplemental bottles, relief bottles, and pacifiers?
- When does he recommend that breast-fed babies start on solid foods, and why? What foods does he recommend be offered first?
- At what age does he recommend that a breast-fed baby be weaned? What method of weaning does he recommend?

PREPARING YOUR BREASTS PRENATALLY

Throughout pregnancy, you can prepare for breastfeeding by practicing good hygiene and using common sense in caring for your breasts. The skin that covers the breast and nipple can be cleansed daily with clear water, and the nipples can be exposed to air and sunlight to help condition the skin. Proper care can eliminate the need for creams and lotions. Colostrum, the yellowish milky substance that is the forerunner of true milk, may occasionally leak from your breasts during pregnancy. This is perfectly normal. Either massage the fluid into your skin or gently wipe it off with clear water. The manual expression of colostrum is not advised since it may open the breast to infection, cause the ductwork to become blocked, or prematurely induce labor.

To prevent the extra weight of the pregnant breast from stretching tissues and eventually causing sagging, a good support bra can be worn during the day. You should, however, avoid bras with tight elastic and underwires, as they can press on milk ducts and decrease circulation. Nursing bras can serve a dual purpose, providing support during pregnancy and lactation and offering the convenience of a front opening for feedings. Choose bras and other clothing that are made of fibers that allow for air circulation and afford maximum absorbency. Cotton is best in both summer and winter, and will help prevent the build-up of moisture that can lead to nipple soreness.

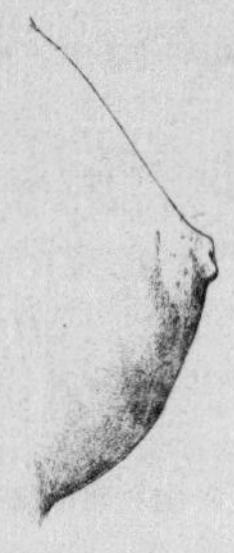

Not Stimulated

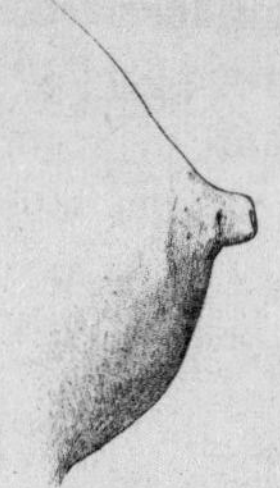

Stimulated

Common Nipple

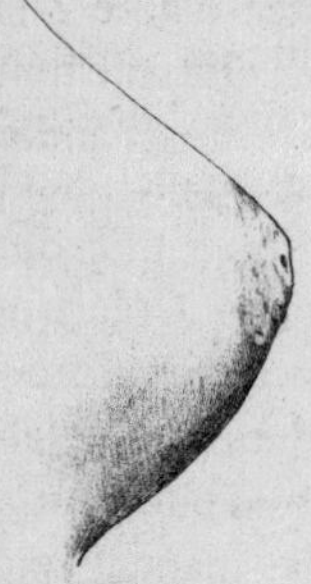

Not Stimulated

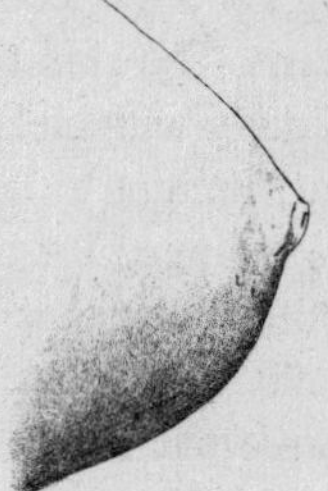

Stimulated

Flat Nipple

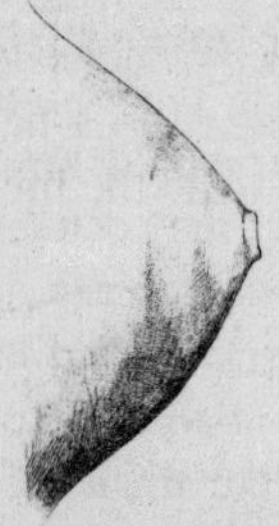

Not Stimulated

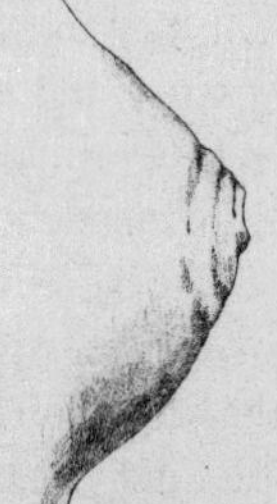

Stimulated

Inverted Nipple

Figure 2.1 Nipple Variations

Correcting Inverted Nipples

One way to prepare your breasts during pregnancy is to check for nipple inversion. About a third of all women have nipples that do not protrude enough to allow their babies to nurse well. Such nipples may be partially or fully inverted. Fortunately, the skin gains elasticity as pregnancy progresses, and only a small percentage of women still have some degree of inversion by their seventh month.

To check for inversion, use your thumb and forefinger to grasp the base of your nipple and press toward the chest wall. Your nipple should become erect. If it withdraws, it is inverted; if it stays the same, it is a flat nipple (see Figure 2.1). If inversion or flatness is still present by the seventh month, begin drawing the nipple out by wearing breast shells and performing the Hoffman technique described below. Most inverted nipples respond well to these techniques; a very small percentage continue to be inverted, requiring patience and work even after delivery.

The Hoffman Technique

This hand technique is recommended by many professionals for improving inverted nipples. To perform the Hoffman technique, place one finger of each hand on opposite sides of the nipple. As shown in Figure 2.2, draw your fingers away from each other, stretching the skin and breaking the small adhesions underneath. Move your fingers around the breast to a new position and repeat the procedure, working all around the breast.

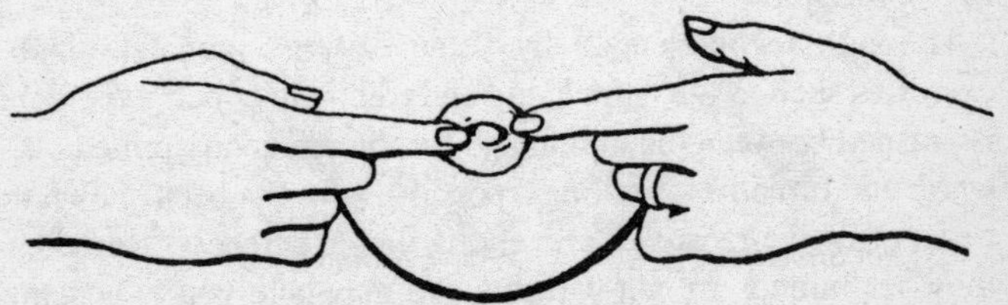

Figure 2.2 Hoffman Technique

Breast Shells

A breast shell, which is also called a breast cup or breast shield, is a dome-shaped plastic cup that has a center opening for the nipple. Breast shells can be worn during the last three months of pregnancy to correct inverted nipples. They work by placing gentle pressure on the base of the nipple, encouraging it to protrude through the shell's opening. Start by wearing the shells for short periods each day, and work up to eight to ten hours a day. By attaching a bra extender to your bra hooks or wearing a larger-sized bra, you will avoid placing excessive pressure on the breasts. Breast shells should never be worn at night or when lying on the breasts, since this may exert undue pressure on breast tissues. See page 220 for a complete discussion of breast shells.

Proper Nipple Care

Even if your nipples do not require corrective techniques, you should prepare for your baby's suckling by taking proper care of the nipple skin. The use of soap and other cleansing agents should be avoided. By removing the natural oils that keep your skin soft and pliable, these substances will increase the likelihood of peeling and cracking.

Since protective layers of skin are developed through pressure on the skin, not friction, you should not rub your nipples in any way. Some professionals recommend rubbing your nipples with a towel as a form of nipple preparation. This practice should be strictly avoided. Rubbing removes the natural oils, wears away the skin, leaves the nipple susceptible to cracking, and is very uncomfortable!

Although recommended by some experts, prenatal nipple exercises such as the "nipple tug and roll"—in which the nipple is grasped between the thumb and forefinger, gently pulled outward, and turned as if rolling a pencil—have not been shown to be an effective means of preventing nipple soreness. However, these techniques are not harmful, and may help you to become more accustomed to handling your breasts.

Breast Massage

Breast massage is encouraged prenatally to increase circulation. In addition, like nipple exercises, massage will help you to become accustomed to handling your breasts. Massage can be practiced in the bath or shower or when you are changing your clothes. Starting from the chest wall under your breast and using the flattened palm of your hand, exert gentle pressure on the breast as you move your hand toward your nipple. Work all around the breast, giving more attention to the areas of greatest duct development, which are under the breast and along the underarm. Once you learn breast massage, you will be able to use it after your baby's birth as a means of inducing relaxation before and during feedings. Refer to page 213 for more information about breast massage.

OTHER WAYS TO PREPARE FOR BREASTFEEDING

In addition to investigating medical services and preparing your breasts for nursing, there are other ways you can get ready for breastfeeding. Consider the practical matters of arranging a nursing corner in your home, planning on the clothing that will make feedings go smoothly, and enlisting the help of family and friends with household chores. To prepare your body for nursing, you should develop an understanding of your nutritional needs during pregnancy and lactation. You should also educate yourself about all aspects of breastfeeding, so that you will have confidence in your ability to nourish your child. The more you learn about and plan for breastfeeding, the more comfortable you will be when it comes time for that first feeding.

Reviewing Your Dietary Practices

When you are pregnant, your doctor will probably provide dietary guidelines that will help to ensure the health of you and your baby. A well-balanced diet with sufficient calories will supply your body with the stores of nutrients you will need to make milk for the first feedings. The more careful you are about the foods you eat during your pregnancy, the better you will feel and the faster you will recover from childbirth. A healthy body is the best form of prevention against illness, postpartum depression, breast infection, and sore nipples.

As a convenient aid to daily food selection, foods are grouped into four categories—milk, meat, fruits and vegetables, and grains—as shown in Table 2.1, The Four Basic Food Groups. Every woman's diet should contain a variety of foods obtained from these four groups. As Table 2.1 indicates, when you are pregnant or lactating, you should eat more servings from most of the groups. You can do this by increasing the amount of foods eaten at each meal and by including two or three nutritious snacks during the day. When your baby begins to eat solid foods, start to cut back on the amount of food you consume so that you will not take in excess calories and begin to gain weight.

The figures in Table 2.1 are all minimum recommended values for the average woman with a normal activity level. If you are more active than most women, increase your nutrients accordingly. Also be aware that women in their teens require more calories, while women aged twenty-five or older require less. Check with your doctor to learn about your personal nutritional requirements.

In order to get the most benefit from the foods you eat, select those foods with the greatest nutritional value. Raw fruits and vegetables, whole grains, and foods that contain the fewest additives and fillers will provide you with the vitamins and minerals your body needs. Choose fresh or frozen foods rather than canned, and use a minimum of heat during their preparation to preserve vitamin content. Prepared foods that contain excess sugar, salt, or fillers will contribute to weight gain without providing the vitamins and minerals vital to your health and the health of your baby. Refer to Chapter 5 for practical meal suggestions and a detailed discussion of diet.

Table 2.1 The Four Basic Food Groups

Food Group (with sample food servings)	**Minimum Recommended Number of Servings Daily**	
	Nonpregnant (1900 calories)	**Pregnant/Lactating (2200 calories)**
Milk or Milk Products 1 cup milk or yogurt. 1½ oz. cheddar cheese. 1 cup pudding. 1¾ cups ice cream. 2 cups cottage cheese. 1 cup tofu (soybean curd).	2	4-5
Meats and Meat Substitutes 2 oz. cooked lean meat, fish, or poultry. 2 oz. cheddar cheese. ½ cup cottage cheese. 1 cup dried beans or peas. 4 tbsp. peanut butter.	2	3-4
Eggs	1	2
Fruits ½ cup cooked or juice. 1 cup raw. 1 medium-sized fruit.	2	3
Vegetables ½ cup cooked. 1 cup raw.	2	4
Grains (whole grain, fortified or enriched) 1 slice bread. 1 cup ready-to-eat cereal. ½ cup cooked cereal, pasta, or grits.	4	4

Preparing Your Home

Making your home a pleasant and convenient place to breastfeed is as important as any other type of breastfeeding preparation. Give some thought to an area in your home where you and your baby can nurse undisturbed. Choose a comfortable armchair and footstool or a reclining chair, and place it either in the bedroom or in another out-of-the-way spot. You can add to your comfort by making several pillows available, and by setting a table or shelf nearby for beverages, snacks, reading materials, and any other items you may need during feedings. Before delivery, you and your mate should plan your baby's sleeping arrangements. In the early weeks, it may be more convenient to have your baby sleep in a crib in your room so that you can easily take him into your bed to nurse at night.

Selecting Clothing and Breastfeeding Supplies

While most clothing for breastfeeding can be adapted from what you already own, you will need to purchase a nursing bra to provide support and facilitate feedings. Select a bra with smooth seams and comfortable straps, avoiding those with tight elastic or underwires that might cause problems by exerting pressure on milk ducts. A bra purchased during the last few months of pregnancy should continue to fit you while you are nursing. Before buying the bra, try it on and check the flaps to see if they can be opened easily with one hand. After purchasing one bra, wear it for a time to see if it is comfortable. If you like it, buy a second one so that you will have a spare.

When preparing for the first few weeks postpartum, the only other items you may need to purchase are two nightgowns that can be easily opened for feedings. Those that button down the front or have elasticized necklines are usually the most convenient. Nursing nightgowns with panels that open under the arm or along the center of the bodice are very nice, but not necessary. During the day, two-piece outfits work well. You can unbutton blouses from the bottom up, leaving the top closed to cover your breasts while your baby covers your abdomen.

When nursing in front of others, drape a sweater, jacket, blanket, poncho, or shawl over your shoulders for additional covering.

The purchase of other items related to breastfeeding—such as breast shells, breast pads, and a breast pump—can be postponed until after your baby arrives. You may never need to use shells or pads, and you probably will not need a pump until your baby is old enough to accept a relief bottle. The exception to this would be if your baby is premature and nursings are delayed.

Planning Household Chores

As you and your baby settle in together, it will be most helpful if you have some assistance with household chores. As a new mother, you will want to spend the majority of your time caring for yourself and your baby. You will need time to get to know your baby, learning his moods and ways. You will also benefit from a stress-free environment in which you can rest, relax, and establish your milk supply. If possible, find someone to care for the household until you can gradually begin to resume your usual duties. Your partner, your mother, or another relative may be able to fill this role. If not, perhaps you can enlist the help of friends to do such chores as shopping, laundry, and meal preparation. Make your arrangements well in advance of your due date. Most important, be sure that everyone understands that you wish to care for your baby and would appreciate help with other tasks. Of course, everyone loves to hold a new baby, and with others around to help with infant care, you will be able to get the rest you need.

Preparing Yourself Mentally

Confidence is the key to successful breastfeeding. By educating yourself about the normal management of breastfeeding, you will discover what to do and what to expect. Learn about how the breast works, familiarize yourself with the various breastfeeding techniques, and gain an understanding of why breast milk is so good for your child. Knowledge of these topics will help you to prevent problems from occurring and will allow you to better enjoy your nursing experience.

By reading this book during pregnancy—and then again after your baby arrives, when you are interested in specific details—you will obtain much of the information you need to succeed. Observing other mothers with their breast-fed babies is another important way of educating yourself. Your local breastfeeding support group can provide you with personal contact with other mothers, as well as giving you many helpful tips. Childbirth classes are another source of breastfeeding information, as are those mothers who have previously nursed children.

While you are educating yourself, share your new knowledge with those close to you. Let your family and friends know that you plan to breastfeed, and help them find answers to their breastfeeding questions before your baby is born. When they understand as much about breastfeeding as you do, they will be more likely to accept your methods of baby care and mothering, and to encourage you to continue breastfeeding.

AT A GLANCE

Planning for Your Baby's Arrival

Selecting Medical Care

- Select a doctor for your baby who will support your decision to breastfeed.
- Learn about hospital or birthing center options, choosing those that will allow for early, frequent feedings.

Preparing Your Body and Mind for Breastfeeding

- Care for your breasts by cleansing them with clear water.
- Use no soaps or breast cremes.
- Wipe off colostrom if it appears, but do not express it.
- To prevent the stretching of tissues that may lead to sagging, wear a good support or nursing bra.
- Check for nipple inversions, using corrective techniques as needed.
- Practice breast massage.
- Eat a balanced diet with sufficient calories.
- Educate yourself, your family, and your friends about breastfeeding.

Preparing for Breastfeeding at Home

- Prepare a nursing corner that is both comfortable and practical.
- Consider sleeping arrangements for your newborn.
- Plan clothing that is suitable for breastfeeding.

Developing a Support System

- Gain the support of friends and relatives.
- Contact a support group.
- Arrange for postpartum help at home.

3
Understanding the Breast

The breast is a fascinating part of the human body. Its beauty and amazing ability to nourish our babies has intrigued mankind for ages. While the way in which the breast works is still not totally understood, much has been learned in recent years. Women now have the advantage of being able to understand how the breasts make milk and how breastfeeding practices can be adapted to meet each baby's needs. By learning about how your breasts function and how breastfeeding management affects that function, you will help to ensure nursing success.

UNDERSTANDING BREAST STRUCTURE

Breast appearance varies greatly from woman to woman. From the large, pendulous bosom to the small, flat breast, the diversity of shapes and sizes is dramatically obvious. This difference is primarily due to the amount of fat in the breast, and is not at all related to the ability to make milk. The tissues responsible for milk production lie deep within the breast, protected by the nonfunctional fatty layer that determines breast size. The nerves within your breast, as well as the skin itself, work in conjunction with these milk-producing tissues in the maintenance of breastfeeding.

The Functional Breast Tissue

Tiny round glands called **alveoli** produce milk in your breasts by selecting nutrients from your blood supply and converting

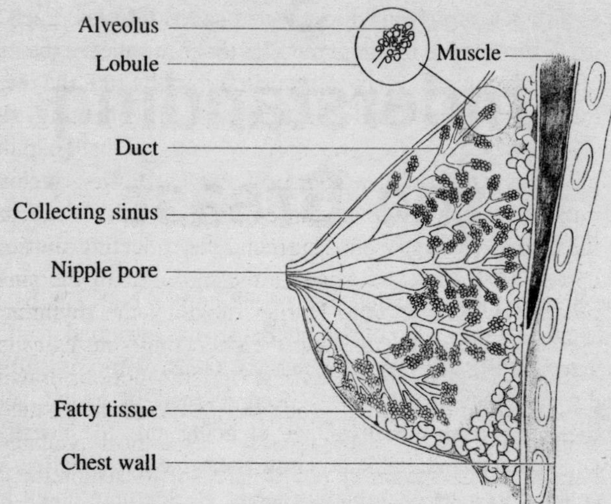

Figure 3.1 Internal Breast Structure

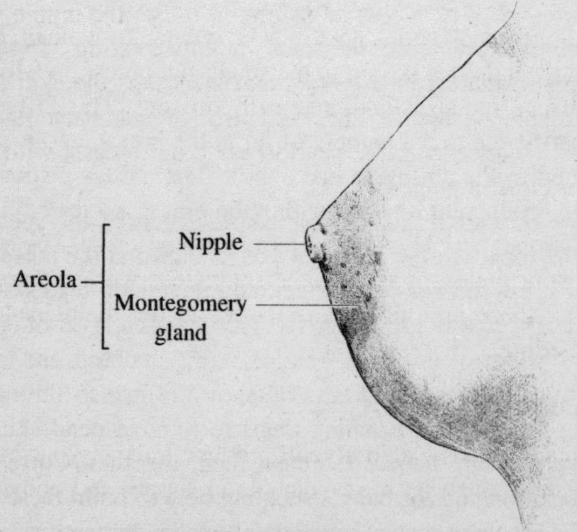

Figure 3.2 The External Breast

them into milk components. These alveoli, which are shown in Figure 3.1, are grouped in clusters called **lobules**. Each alveolus is surrounded by small muscles that can squeeze the milk out of the alveolus and into tubes called **ducts**. From the ducts, the milk moves into enlarged tubes called **collecting sinuses**. There, the milk is held in reserve by muscles that keep the nipple pores closed. When your baby nurses, he first receives the milk from the collecting sinuses. If his mouth is well back on the breast so that his gums surround the collecting sinuses, he is able to both suck and squeeze the milk out of the sinuses, a process called **suckling**. During suckling, the rhythmic compression of his gums around the collecting sinuses causes the walls of the ducts to move in a rippling motion, drawing the milk from the alveoli. If your baby's mouth is on the nipple alone, however, he is able to suck out the most available milk, but cannot draw the milk out of the ducts to sustain the flow.

The Skin and Nerves of the Breast

When your baby sees your breast, he is most aware of the nipple and the darkened skin around it, called the **areola** (see Figure 3.2). The areola helps him to locate the nipple visually. Within the areola are the small, pimply-looking **Montgomery glands**, which secrete a fluid that lubricates the skin covering the nipple and areola. This fluid also prevents bacterial growth, thereby eliminating the need to wash the breasts with soap or other cleansing agents.

The skin around the nipple and areola is of the special type that is found on the palms of your hands and the soles of your feet. It has the ability to retain outer layers of dead skin, forming a tough, waterproof barrier. This callused layer of dead cells helps protect your nipple from soreness, cracking, and infection. Contrary to popular belief, calluses are formed through pressure, not friction. Rubbing tends to remove dead skin layers, while pressure helps to cement them together. Correct breast preparation and the baby's suckling help to build these layers.

The areola is special in another way. Underneath it lie nerves that, while unaffected by light touch, are stimulated by the strong pressure of your baby's gums. When your baby clamps down on the areola to suckle the milk out of the collecting sinuses, he stimulates deep nerves that send signals to your brain, initiating milk production and milk release. It is important that your baby be positioned well back on the areola for three reasons: to stimulate the deep nerves in order to trigger milk production and release, to efficiently remove milk from the collecting sinuses, and to ensure that the nipple is not made sore by the stress of your baby nursing on the end of it.

BREAST CHANGES BEFORE AND DURING PREGNANCY

Noticeable breast development begins in puberty, and is augmented by the hormones released during the first menstrual cycle. Monthly hormonal changes cause the growth of ducts and other tissues, while a thick layer of fat is deposited under the skin to form the spherical adolescent breast. Each time an egg is released from the ovaries, the breast starts to retain fluids. This furthers the development of ducts and alveoli in preparation for pregnancy. When pregnancy does not occur, this growth partially regresses, but the breast never returns to its previous state. Thus, breast development is enhanced with each menstrual period.

Changes in the First Trimester

With conception, hormonal changes cause the breast to develop dramatically (see Figure 3.3). During the **first trimester** (0-3 months), the ducts multiply, the Montgomery glands enlarge, and the skin of the areola and nipple darkens. The Montgomery glands begin secreting the protective, oily lubricant that will continue to be produced throughout pregnancy and lactation. You may notice some soreness or tenderness in your breasts as the tissues develop and the skin stretches.

Changes in the Second Trimester

During the **second trimester** (4-6 months), the duct system continues to branch and grow, while alveoli begin to develop in preparation for milk production. At about four months, colostrum production begins. Colostrum is a highly nutritious, thick, yellowish fluid that is perfectly suited to the newborn baby's needs. By six months, there is sufficient breast development to provide adequate amounts of colostrum and milk to sus-

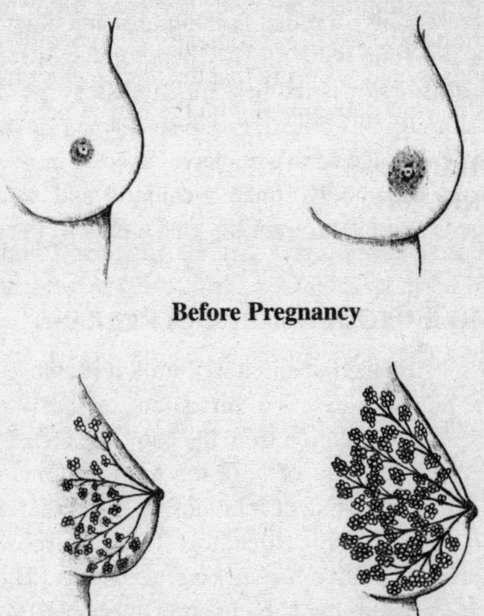

During Pregnancy

Note the enlarged areola and increased milk-producing tissue.

Figure 3.3 Breast Changes During Pregnancy

tain a newborn; if the baby were born that early, breastfeeding would be possible. Although the hormones of pregnancy suppress its secretion, colostrum sometimes leaks out of the nipple pores, especially late in the pregnancy. Because of the development and growth of the alveoli and the expanded volume of blood and other fluids in the breast, the weight of the breast increases by one to one and a half pounds during this trimester.

Changes in the Third Trimester

With increased breast development in the **third trimester** (7-9 months), breast skin may become stressed and stretch marks may appear. There are no creams or lotions that can remove stretch marks; however, they usually vanish several months after birth. Breast size generally stabilizes during this period, so you can be reasonably sure that nursing bras and other clothing purchased at this time will still fit when you begin breastfeeding. The third trimester is the best time to assess the degree of nipple inversion. By this time, the skin has gained elasticity, and only a small percentage of women have inverted nipples. These women should use the Hoffman technique and wear breast shells to increase nipple protractility (the ability of the nipple to protrude).

BREAST MILK PRODUCTION AND RELEASE

Considering its size and the amount of milk it is able to produce each day, the human breast is a miraculous organ. With proper care and adequate stimulation from the baby, the breast will produce precisely the amount of milk the baby requires to thrive and grow. The interdependent relationship of mother and baby is the key to successful breastfeeding. The baby must be nurtured, nourished, and have his sucking needs met. The mother yearns to nurture, needs her baby to empty her breasts to relieve fullness, and requires nipple stimulation for milk production. In a relaxed atmosphere, without interference, the mother-baby team functions well for the mother who is knowledgeable about both her needs and those of her baby.

How Milk Production Begins

Throughout pregnancy, your breasts develop milk-producing tissues in readiness for your baby's first nursing. Simultaneously, your body increases the levels of **prolactin**, the hormone that causes milk to be produced. By term, prolactin levels are very high but are suppressed by high levels of two other hormones, **estrogen** and **progesterone**. As soon as the placenta is delivered, the levels of estrogen and progesterone in your body drop dramatically. This signals the alveoli in your breasts to begin making milk. The method of delivery—vaginal or Cesarean—is unrelated to your body's ability to begin making milk. Delivery of the placenta is the trigger that begins the process of milk production.

Your Supply of Breast Milk

The amount of milk produced by your breasts depends on the level of the hormone prolactin in your body. After rising to a peak at birth, your body's prolactin level gradually decreases for several weeks after delivery. However, each time you nurse and your baby stimulates the nerves in your nipples, the prolactin level rises to ten times the base level. Therefore, the frequency of nursing directly controls milk production: the more your baby nurses, the more milk you will produce. On the other hand, practices that interfere with nipple stimulation—the use of a nipple shield, a rigid four-hour feeding schedule, or the use of supplemental bottles—will decrease milk production. If you nurse as often as your baby needs feeding, your milk supply will continually increase to meet his requirements. In the first weeks, nursing at least nine times in twenty-four hours has been found to be most conducive to the establishment of an adequate milk supply. This direct link between nursing and milk production explains why women with large babies, twins, or even triplets can produce enough milk to satisfy their babies.

Table 3.1 indicates the average amount of breast milk that is produced each day at various stages of your baby's development. Depending on your baby's size and his nursing pattern, these quantities will vary. The maximum amount utilized will be about one quart a day between two and six months of age. Babies on formula sometimes require more than this, as formula is not as completely digested and utilized by the body. Formula-fed babies also require additional fluids, such as water, to remove unused minerals. Because the digestion of breast milk produces fewer waste products, breast-fed babies require no supplemental fluids.

Table 3.1 Average Amounts of Breast Milk Produced

Baby's Age (months)	Quantity (ounces/day)
Newborn	20.3
1	26.5
2	28.4
6	27.8
6-12	18.6
12-24	15.2

Several other factors may affect your milk supply. A poor diet can reduce your ability to produce milk. Inadequate emptying of the breast or a failure to let down the milk will cause milk to accumulate, putting pressure on milk-producing tissues and decreasing their output. Consequently, it is very important to nurse on one breast until the baby signals the end of the feeding on that breast by releasing the nipple.

The Letdown of Your Milk

When your baby suckles at your breast, he not only stimulates milk to be produced, but also causes the milk to be expelled (see Figure 3.4). As a result of suckling, the hormone **oxytocin** is released, causing the contraction of the small muscles around the milk-producing cells and squeezing milk down into the ducts, where your baby can remove it. The expulsion of milk down the ducts, called **letdown**, occurs several times during each feeding. Tension, anxiety, pain, fear, and excitement can block oxytocin from doing its job, so that only the milk already in the collecting sinuses is available to your baby. This means that he can only obtain a third of the milk while the other two thirds remain in your breasts.

To ensure good letdowns throughout each of the early feed-

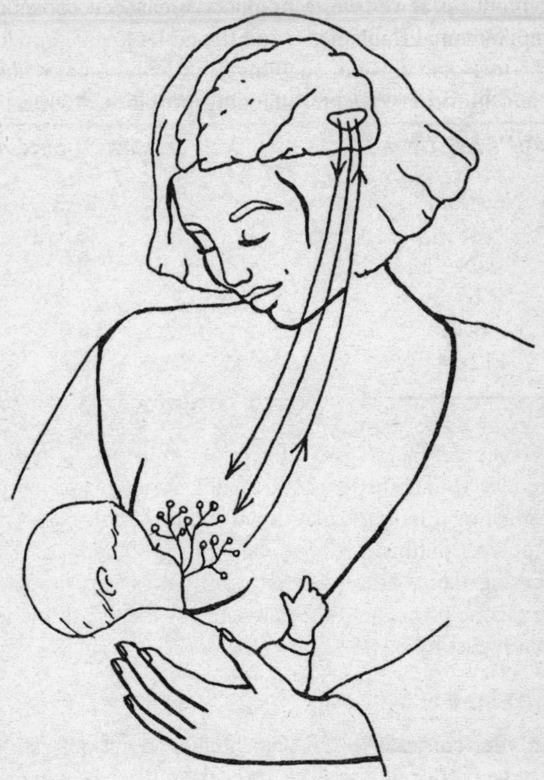

Figure 3.4 Pathways of Milk Production and Release

ings, try to relax while nursing. Once your letdown has been established, you can psychologically condition your milk to be released by repeating familiar patterns. A comfortable chair, pillows, a beverage, and a quiet place to nurse will all help. The use of breast massage prior to nursing is also very effective. In addition, you may want to take some deep breaths, or to visualize your milk flowing. Fortunately, one of the side effects of nursing is a feeling of relaxation, so most women have no problem with letdown. In fact, you may find that simply picking your baby up or hearing him cry will cause your milk to let down. A firmly established, conditioned letdown can withstand much stress and tension, enabling your baby to enjoy the comfort and nutrition that breastfeeding provides despite the ups and downs of daily life.

AT A GLANCE

Understanding the Breast

Breast Structure

- Breast size is determined by the amount of fat contained in the breast and has no bearing on the ability to make milk.
- Tiny alveolar glands make milk in the breast.
- Milk is held in the collecting sinuses beneath the areola.
- Nerves within the nipple and areola must be stimulated for milk to be produced and released.
- Montgomery glands secrete a protective lubricating fluid on the skin of the areola and nipple, eliminating the need for cleansing with soap.
- Callused layers of skin formed by pressure, not friction, protect the nipple skin from being broken down.

Breast Development and Milk Production

- Breast development begins at puberty, and continues with each menstrual cycle.
- Pregnancy causes a rapid growth of the breast tissues.
- Colostrum production begins during the fourth month of pregnancy.
- By 6 months after conception, the breast is sufficiently developed to secrete enough colostrum and milk to sustain life in the event of premature birth.
- Delivery of the placenta causes milk production to begin.

Your Supply of Breast Milk

- The more often you nurse, the more milk you produce.
- In the first few weeks, nurse at least 9 times in each 24-hour period to ensure a plentiful milk supply.
- To stimulate your breasts and maintain milk production, nurse on each breast until your baby signals that no more milk is available by releasing the nipple from his mouth.
- Use relaxtion techniques to ensure good letdowns so that all of the milk in your breasts is made available to your baby.

4

Breast Milk and Your Baby

Nursing will not only offer the warmth and security of your presence to your baby, but will also provide him with the best food available: breast milk. Always ready and at the perfect temperature, breast milk contains all the nutrients your baby will need in exactly the right proportions for growth at each stage of his development. Your nursing baby will also be protected against many illnesses by receiving your milk. Thus, breast milk offers a double health benefit to your baby: excellent nutrition and disease protection. Keeping your milk free of drugs, alcohol, and other contaminants will help ensure that your baby receives the best possible nutrition.

THE UNIQUE PROPERTIES OF HUMAN MILK

An ever-changing fluid, breast milk is almost magical in nature. Its composition will alter throughout each day, as well as each feeding, to meet your baby's needs. A watery, high-carbohydrate mixture will be present in the morning when your baby is alert, while a richer, fattier milk will be available in the afternoon and evening as your baby is readied for sleep. Milk will even adapt to your environment, producing live cells and antibodies in response to many diseases to which you are exposed. In addition to these qualities, human milk has a very low bacteria count, as well as elements that discourage spoilage. Although you may think that breast milk is similar to formula, the differences are dramatic. While formula is consistently the same, never varying from bottle to bottle, no two feedings of breast milk are alike. Your milk is as alive and vital as the blood circulating in your body!

Colostrum

What is yellowish, thicker than mature milk, and contains many times more antibodies? It is **colostrum**, the earliest form of human milk, which provides the newborn with the immunities his body needs to fight off disease. Colostrum also acts as a laxative to clean **meconium** (the first stools of the newborn) out of his system and to aid his body in ridding itself of waste products. Secreted from the breasts after delivery, colostrum begins mixing with true milk in the second or third day and totally disappears after about ten days. When you offer colostrum to your baby, you will be giving him the best nutritional start he can get.

True Breast Milk

What is watery, looks bluish white, comes preheated, and is full of nutrients, antibodies, and live cells? The answer is the most perfect food for your infant: human milk. Even after the transition from colostrum to true breast milk, human milk never looks like cow's milk or formula. Breast milk is much thinner and is not homogenized, which is why it separates when left to stand. The color may appear bluish, greenish, or even yellowish, depending on your own diet and vitamin supplements. This unfamiliar appearance may cause you to think that your milk is weak or harmful to your baby. On the contrary, it is ideally suited to your baby's growth rate, just as cow's milk is suited to the faster growth rate of a newborn calf.

The first milk that your baby will obtain at each feeding—**foremilk**—is especially thin and watery, with a high protein and carbohydrate content. That is why expressed or pumped milk may appear deceptively thin. Milk obtained at the end of the feeding is much higher in calories, most of which come from fat particles. Up to one half of the calories in breast milk are obtained from this fatty **hindmilk**. It is important that you let your baby nurse long enough at each breast— until he releases the nipple spontaneously—to obtain the calories he needs to thrive.

Nutrient Components of Breast Milk

Human milk is a complex solution of carbohydrates, fats, and proteins. The composition varies from one woman to another, from week to week, and even from hour to hour. The balance of carbohydrates, fats, and proteins is precisely suited to the infant's growth at each stage of his development. The mineral content of breast milk is very stable and relatively independent of your diet, with stores in your body supplying what your diet lacks. The fat-soluble vitamins—A, D, E, and K—vary little from one milk sample to the next; however, water-soluble vitamins, such as Vitamin C and all of the B vitamins, depend on your daily intake. Since water-soluble vitamins are not stored well by the body, they need to be replaced at each meal. Fresh fruits and vegetables provide an abundance of all of these vitamins except for Vitamin B12, which can be obtained from red meats, fish, eggs, milk, and cheese.

Vitamin and Mineral Supplements for Your Baby

Because human milk contains all necessary nutrients in ideal proportions for your baby's growth and development, vitamin and mineral supplements are not usually needed. In the past, it was believed that breast milk contained inadequate amounts of Vitamin D and iron. However, recent research has shown that more Vitamin D is present than was previously believed.[1] Also, Vitamin D can be obtained by exposing the skin to sunlight. Thirty minutes of exposure will satisfy the weekly requirements of a light-skinned baby. The baby should be fully clothed, but should not be wearing a hat. Dark-skinned babies require longer periods of exposure.[2] The effect of the sunlight, along with the nutrients contained in your breast milk, will provide your infant with an ample supply of Vitamin D.

Although breast milk contains only small amounts of iron, the iron is in a form that enables it to be completely utilized by the baby. Other components of the milk enhance iron absorption, so that full-term breastfed babies do not normally require iron supplementation.[3] Premature babies, and those who did not receive the full complement of iron in utero, do require supplements. Routine iron supplementation is not advised, however, since it interferes with elements in the milk that decrease the amount of tooth decay bacteria in the mouth.[4] Excess iron can also cause an increase of certain intestinal bacteria, resulting in digestive disorders.[5] Naturally, supplements should never be given to your child without medical supervision.

The need for supplementing your baby's diet with fluoride is presently a center of controversy. Fluoride supplements have been shown to decrease infant tooth decay by 50 to 60 percent. When a breastfeeding mother ingests fluoride, small amounts appear in her milk, but it is believed that the quantites are too small to prevent tooth decay. On the other hand, some mothers report that their infants are allergic to fluoride, or that supplements cause digestive upsets. In addition, excessive doses of fluoride can cause discoloration of the teeth, and it is difficult to assess exactly how much fluoride an infant is receiving. The American Academy of Pediatrics recommends that fluoride supplements be started shortly after birth, but also recognizes that supplementation can be delayed for six months.[6] You and your baby's doctor may wish to start your baby on fluoride in the early weeks and watch him for any reactions. If fussiness, irritability, or spitting up occurs, consider the possibility of discontinuing the fluoride supplements until your child is six months of age.

Protective Components of Breast Milk

Breast milk contains many ingredients beyond the basic nutrients. Within your milk, live cells engulf and digest bacteria, and also produce antibodies to bacteria. Special components enhance the absorption of other nutrients and establish conditions in your baby's mouth and digestive system that discourage bacterial growth. Your milk will provide your baby with antibodies to many of the diseases to which you have been exposed. In addition, when you are ill, your milk will often help protect your baby from that particular disease. Therefore, you can usually nurse your baby even when you are sick, provided that you are not too weak to manage and that you are not taking any medication that may harm him. To avoid unnecessary exposure, take the precaution of limiting mouth and nose contact, and wash your hands before caring for your baby.

Breast milk can help reduce the incidence of allergies in babies. First, it delays the onset of allergies by taking the place of foods to which your baby may be sensitive. Second, breast milk helps cover the small openings in your baby's intestine through which foreign proteins from foods can pass. By feeding your baby breast milk exclusively and delaying the introduction of solid foods until he is six months of age, you will limit your baby's exposure to potentially allergenic (allergy-producing) foods until his system is sufficiently mature to handle them, and will thus decrease his chances of developing food sensitivities. When your baby is two years old, he should be able to handle all foods, including those that most commonly cause allergic reactions.

IMPURITIES THAT CAN ENTER YOUR BREAST MILK

While breast milk is usually thought of as being pure, the breast cannot completely filter out all foreign substances. Some components of the foods you ingest, the medicines you take, and the air you breathe will end up in your milk. Although most of these elements will not harm your baby, some products and practices should be avoided to prevent him from receiving an excessive amount of offending substances.

Medications

The best rule in regard to medications is to avoid them as much as possible. When you must take a drug, avoid long-acting preparations, and use the smallest dosage in the form that is least harmful to your baby. Even over-the-counter products like aspirin and cold remedies should be avoided unless absolutely necessary—and then should be taken only with the knowledge of your baby's doctor. While the strength of some ingredients will be greatly diminished by the time they reach your breast milk, others will be more concentrated in your milk than they are in your blood stream. Certain products, like antihistamines, will not only enter your milk, but may also reduce your milk output. Whenever a doctor prescribes any medication for you, be sure to let him know that you are nursing so that he can select the safest possible product. If you are under treatment for a chronic condition, your doctor may be able to prescribe a drug that is compatible with nursing. If you notice that a drug is affecting your baby or your milk supply in any way, stop taking it and request that your doctor provide an alternative treatment.

The activity of some drugs is very short-lived, so you may be able to alter your feeding times or skip a feeding to prevent your baby from ingesting a large dose. For ongoing health problems, treatment may sometimes be delayed until your baby is older. If none of these alternatives is open to you, a suspension of breastfeeding may be necessary, depending on your baby's age and weight and on the other foods in his diet. In any case, you and your doctor must decide whether the benefit to you outweighs any possible risks to your baby.

Social Drugs

When you realize the harm that may be caused by prescription and over-the-counter medications, it quickly becomes apparent that social drugs such as marijuana, amphetamines, heroin, and cocaine should be *strictly avoided*. These drugs can interfere with your ability to care for your baby. They can also cause behavioral changes and permanent damage in your baby. Depressants can result in sleepiness, decreased appetite, and the inability to suckle, leading to undernutrition. Marijuana reaches the baby through breast milk in levels capable of causing structural changes in his brain cells and impairing growth. If you are now using any of these drugs, you should either make every effort to stop immediately or recognize that you cannot safely nurse your baby.

Nicotine

Because impurities can enter your milk through the air you breathe, it is wise to avoid all toxic fumes, including cigarette smoke. Excessive amounts of nicotine in your breast milk can cause nausea and vomiting in your baby. By using up your stores of Vitamin C, smoking may decrease the Vitamin C content of your milk. In addition, smoking may interfere with breastfeeding by preventing your milk from letting down and by decreasing your milk supply.

The effects of nicotine in milk are minor, however, when compared with the effects of smoke inhalation. Your baby can ingest much more nicotine directly from smoke in the air than he can from your milk, and the resultant tars in his lungs will increase his susceptibility to colds and other respiratory diseases.

If at all possible, stop smoking when breastfeeding. If you cannot stop, try to cut down. If you continue to smoke while lactating, consider increasing your intake of Vitamin C to ensure that your infant will receive an adequate amount. In addition, take precautions to avoid exposing your baby to cigarette smoke—whether it's a result of your own smoking or that of others.

Alcohol

At some time during the nursing relationship, you may be confronted with the question of how social drinking might affect the health of your infant. In the past, nursing mothers were often encouraged to drink one glass of beer or wine in order to relax. With the possibility that misinterpretation could occur and the mother drink more than a moderate amount, such recommendations are no longer made.

Alcohol, like most other substances, does enter breast milk.

The level of alcohol in your milk will be the same as that in your blood stream, a level that can be harmful to an infant, whose immature system makes him more susceptible than an adult to alcohol's effects. In addition, large amounts of alcohol may block your letdown reflex and interfere with your ability to care for your child.

For the mother, the effects of drinking are most pronounced within the first two hours, and taper off as the alcohol passes through your body. However, the alcohol level in the blood stream and milk drops off slowly, and significant traces are still present six hours after consuming one drink. Moreover, although drinking after eating reduces the visible effects of alcohol consumption, the presence of food in the stomach does not prevent the alcohol from eventually reaching the milk.

If you choose to drink, try to limit yourself to small amounts, and temporarily discontinue nursing for four to six hours afterwards. In order to ensure that your baby will not receive a significant amount of alcohol, express and discard your milk before nursing.

Environmental Pollutants

Periodically, the news media have carried stories about the contamination of breast milk by environmental pollutants. While pollutants such as DDT, PCB, and PBB have been identified in some milk samples, there is no evidence of their harmful effects on babies. Any risks to your baby resulting from your normal daily exposure will be far outweighed by the many benefits of breast milk.

It is the mother's diet and nutritional status that determine whether the pollutants contained in her body are transmitted to her breast milk. Toxic substances are stored in human fat. They are released when the body's energy supply is depleted and fat is needed to provide additional energy. In a well-nourished woman, only small amounts of body fat are utilized in milk production. Malnutrition or rapid weight loss, however, can release the pollutants that are stored in the body's fat, producing higher levels in the mother's milk.

To make sure that your milk is as pure as possible, reduce the risks of exposure and limit the amount of pollutants you ingest and inhale. Do not use household sprays, especially pesticides, and do not eat freshwater fish from potentially polluted waters. Cut off the fat (where pollutants are stored) from meats prior to cooking, and wash or peel fruits and vegetables. Avoid jobs that expose you to lead, cadmium, mercury, or plastic-type chemicals, and avoid mothproofed clothing containing dieldrin. In addition, maintain a proper diet and avoid excessive weight loss in order to prevent the toxic substances stored in your body from being released and entering your breast milk.

By feeding your baby breast milk that is as free as possible of pollutants and drugs, you will gain peace of mind, and your baby will receive the best possible food. Your milk will protect him from many illnesses and help to prevent infantile allergies and colic. Without the setbacks that accompany these problems, you and your baby will have more time to enjoy each other and to benefit from the special closeness and warmth that only breastfeeding can provide.

AT A GLANCE

Breast Milk and Your Baby

Characteristics of Breast Milk

- Human milk does not look like cow's milk; it is thin and bluish in color.
- Colostrum, the forerunner of true milk, is the best available form of newborn nutrition.
- Milk composition varies during each feeding, as well as from hour to hour, day to day, and woman to woman.
- The relative quantities of nutrients in milk are ideally suited to your baby's needs.
- Breast milk contains disease-protective factors.
- Breast milk contains components that will reduce or delay allergic reactions in your baby.

Keeping Your Breast Milk Pure

- Provided that you practice good hygiene, illness should not usually prevent you from nursing.
- Avoid all medications when possible.
- Avoid all social drugs.
- When drugs are necessary, select forms and nursing times that will minimize the medication's effects on your baby.
- Cut down on cigarette smoking as much as possible, and avoid exposing your baby to smoke.
- Keep alcoholic drinks to a minimum, and do not nurse after consuming large amounts of alcohol.
- Decrease enviornmental contaminants in your milk by avoiding exposure to pollutants and by postponing the loss of significant amounts of weight until the baby has been weaned.

5

Eating Well for You and Your Baby

While many of us are aware of the basic rules for a sound diet, few give nutrition much thought in our daily lives. During pregnancy, however, women often begin to wonder just what effect their eating has on the fetus, and consequently develop a new interest in nutrition. Similarly, as long as you breastfeed your child, food selection and eating patterns will be a means of ensuring the health of your baby.

MEETING YOUR NUTRITIONAL NEEDS WHILE NURSING

In order to nurse successfully, you will need to eat the same type of balanced diet that you did while you were pregnant. If your baby exhibits an allergic reaction to any food in your diet, it will be necessary to avoid that food. However, most women can eat the foods they enjoy without causing their babies any distress. Food selection need not be difficult or time consuming. The sampling of new foods may provide unexpected dividends for you and your family in terms of a lifetime of healthful eating. The key to wise food selection is coordinating the foods available to you in each season with your budget, your preferences, and your body's needs.

Counting Calories

Until recently, it was thought that a lactating woman required a greater number of calories than a pregnant woman. However, a 1986 study showed that a woman's metabolism is more efficient during lactation than at any other time, and that she requires fewer calories than previously recommended.[1] You will need approximately 2,200 calories to produce enough milk for your baby while maintaining your health.[2] If you are underweight, undernourished, nursing more than one baby, or very active, you will require even more calories. Simply by adding healthful snacks to your diet, you will obtain the extra calories and nutrients you need. For example, a snack of peanut butter and jelly on two slices of whole wheat bread and an eight-ounce glass of milk will provide you with 500 calories.

Drinking Sufficient Fluids

Because milk is 87 percent water, your fluid intake will be important while nursing. An average of six to eight cups of liquid each day should be sufficient to meet your needs. Forcing fluids is not necessary. Just drink to satisfy your thirst—an easy requirement to fulfill, since nursing makes you very thirsty! If you do not drink enough liquids, you may notice that your skin and lips become dry, or you may have a problem with constipation. One way to make sure you get enough fluids is to drink something each time you nurse. You will automatically be replacing lost fluids, and the simple act of drinking may help to condition your letdown. Water, pure, unsweetened fruit juices, and milk are the best beverages for the nursing mother.

Improving Your Diet

Although most women realize that they should improve their eating habits, they often lack the incentive to do so. Caring for a new baby and breastfeeding may provide you with the motivation to explore more healthful ways of eating. Producing plenty of high-quality milk requires a nutritious diet, and caring for a baby takes considerable energy. Poor eating habits are often the result of a lack of planning, and improvement may be as easy as developing a weekly meal plan and writing out a shopping list.

Set a goal of eating three balanced meals and two or three nutritious snacks a day. Focus on eliminating those dietary practices that you feel are least desirable, for example, skipping breakfast, snacking on soda and chips, or passing up vegetables. As you improve your diet, you may begin to realize how much good food you can eat without gaining weight.

Gradual changes that fit into your lifestyle and circumstances are the easiest to manage. As your baby grows, you may want to investigate other ways of improving your family's diet. You can replace refined flours with whole grain products, substitute fresh and frozen foods for canned, and eliminate highly processed foods that contain additives.

Eating a variety of foods will help ensure that your diet contains foods from all four groups. In addition, by selecting fruits and vegetables from various parts of the plants—stems (celery), leaves (spinach), fruit (tomato), and roots (carrots)—you will obtain a good balance of vitamins and minerals. It is especially important to obtain extra calcium while you are nursing. If your calcium intake is low, calcium for your milk will be taken from your body, leaving your bones depleted. This may cause your bones to weaken or even fracture in later years.

While nursing, your body will require 1,200 milligrams (mg) of calcium each day. This increase of 400 mg over what you needed before you became pregnant can be obtained from eleven ounces of milk. If you prefer not to drink milk, you can obtain sufficient calcium from other sources such as cheese, yogurt, and greens. As shown by Table 5.1, there are many different sources of calcium you can incorporate into your diet. If you are unable to get enough calcium from your foods, you may wish to take calcium supplements. Calcium should always be

Table 5.1 Good Sources of Calcium

Food	Calcium (mgs per servings)	Supplements
Yogurt, plain (8 oz.)	415	Because many women do not eat enough calcium-rich foods, many experts recommend calcium supplements. Calcium gluconate and calcium lactate are the safest supplements. We advise against taking bone meal because several brands contain high levels of lead. Dolomite is also a poor choice because it may contain lead or other toxic metals.
Cheddar cheese (2 oz.)	408	
Sardines, drained (3 oz.)	372	
Milk, skim or lowfat protein-fortified (8 oz.)	352	
American cheese (2 oz.)	348	
Yogurt, fruit flavored (8 oz.)	345	
Milk, whole, lowfat or skim (8 oz.)	297	
Watercress (1 cup chopped)	189	
Chocolate pudding, instant (1/2 cup)	187	
Collards (1/2 cup cooked)	179	
Buttermilk pancakes (3-4")	174	
Pink salmon, canned (3 oz.)	167	
Tofu (4 oz.)	145	Experts say that there are no significant side effects from taking a supplement of between 500 and and 1,000 milligrams of calcium per day. Only in people with sarcoidosis or a few other diseases can this amount of calcium cause problems.
Turnip greens (1/2 cup cooked)	134	
Kale (1/2 cup cooked)	103	
Shrimp, canned (3 oz.)	99	
Ice cream (1/2 cup)	88	
Okra (1/2 cup cooked)	74	
Rutabaga,mashed (1/2 cup cooked)	71	
Broccoli (1/2 cup cooked)	68	
Soybeans (1/2 cup cooked)	66	
Cottage cheese (1/2 cup)	63	
Bread, white or whole wheat (2 sl.)	48	

Reprinted from Nutrition Action Healthletter, which is available from the Center for Science in the Public Interest, 1501 16th Street, N.W., Washington, D.C. 20036, for $20.00 per year, copyright 1986.

taken in combination with Vitamin D so that your body is better able to use it. Check with your doctor for the type and dosage that will meet your specific needs.

Reducing Food Costs

Dietary improvement does not have to be expensive. The increased cost of purchasing fresh fruits and vegetables can be offset by the elimination of high-priced processed foods. Convenience foods are often expensive because of the packaging. By using basic ingredients, you can prepare the same thing for a lot less money—and in not much more time. For example, dry packaged mixes only save you the time of measuring out the ingredients; the balance of the process is the same no matter which way you prepare the food. Most important, by using ingredients from your kitchen, you will avoid fillers, preservatives, and other additives.

You can significantly cut down on your food costs by planning meals to minimize waste, sticking to your shopping list, reading labels, purchasing sale items, utilizing meat substitutes, and purchasing less expensive cuts of meat. Table 5.2 provides suggestions for a wide variety of meatless casseroles that are very inexpensive and easy to make. As a breastfeeding mother, you may be eligible for nutrition assistance from the food program for Women, Infants and Children (WIC). As long as you plan wisely and maintain your spirit of adventure, improving your diet can be both economical and enjoyable. The benefits to your health will be well worth the effort.

If you are a working mother or if you lead a busy social life, you probably eat out fairly often. In order to get the best nutrition for your dollar, you should select such foods as salads, soups, fish, and chicken, all of which generally contain less fat than other entrees. You may find that the weekend is a convenient time to do a large portion of the week's meal preparation, allowing you to make several meals at once and store them in the refrigerator or freezer. If you prefer to purchase convenience foods, avoid salt, sugars, fats, and fillers, and look for those products with a high protein content. When possible, make use of such conveniences as the Crock-Pot electric cooker, the microwave oven, and pre-timed oven cooking. These can save time and help you fit meal preparation into your schedule.

Foods to Avoid

Most women can continue to eat their favorite dishes while nursing. However, there may be times when you will need to cut down on certain foods. Occasionally, spicy foods or those in the cabbage family can give a baby indigestion or gas. Do not feel that you must automatically avoid such foods. Just eat whatever you enjoy in moderation and watch your baby for signs of discomfort, eliminating only those items that definitely cause an adverse reaction. Your baby will probably enjoy the flavors of those highly aromatic foods that come through your milk, and this exposure may help him become accustomed to new tastes.

Some babies are sensitive to caffeine and may react to it by becoming irritable, wakeful, and difficult to calm. If you notice any of these signs in your baby, it would be wise to cut down on coffee, tea, chocolate, cola, and all medications that contain caffeine. In extreme cases, it may be necessary for you to totally avoid caffeine for several months, until your baby's system matures. The caffeine content of a number of foods is presented in Table 5.3.

Although it sometimes seems that a baby is allergic to his own mother's milk, this has never been shown to be the case. Allergic reactions—including gas, diarrhea, spitting up, vomiting, colic, and skin rash—usually occur because the baby is sensitive to some food eaten by his mother, especially when this food is eaten in excess. Such reactions occur more frequently when there is a family history of allergies. Eating a well-balanced diet with reasonable amounts of a variety of foods usually eliminates this problem.

The food that is most likely to cause an allergic reaction is cow's milk. In one study, three quarters of the women who eliminated all forms of cow's milk from their diets saw the allergic

Table 5.2 Complete Protein Casseroles

Choose one ingredient from each of the five columns below. Mix together ingredients from the first four columns. Pour into greased casserole dish (2 quart) and bake 30 minutes at 375°F. Top with one choice from column five and bake 15 minutes longer at 325°F. Salt to taste at the table. Serve with bread and a salad.

Grain: 2 cups cooked	**Beans:** 1 cups cooked	**Sauce:** 1 can soup & ¾ cup water	**Vegetables:** to make 1 ½ cups	**Toppings:** to make 3-5 tablespoons
Brown Rice.	Soybeans.	Cream of tomato soup.	Browned celery & green onions.	Wheatgerm.
Macaroni, enriched or whole wheat.	Dried lima beans.	Cream of potato soup.	Mushroom and bamboo shoots.	Slivered almonds.
Corn.	Dried whole or split peas.	Cream of Mushroom soup.	Browned green pepper & garlic.	Fresh whole wheat bread crumbs.
Spagetti, enriched or whole wheat.	Kidney beans.	Cream of celery soup.	Cooked green beans.	Sesame seeds.
White rice, converted.	Lentils.	Cheddar cheese soup.	Cooked carrots.	Chopped peanuts.
Noodles, enriched or whole wheat.	Garbanzos (chickpeas).	Cream of pea soup.	Browned onion & pimento.	Sunflower seeds.

Table 5.3 The Common Sources of Caffeine

Product	Caffeine (in milligrams)
Coffee (5 oz.)	
Brewed, drip method	115
Brewed, percolator	80
Instant	65
Decaffeinated, brewed	3
Decaffeinated, instant	2
Tea (5 oz.)	
Brewed, major U.S. brands	40
Brewed, important brands	60
Instant	30
Iced (12 oz.)	70
Soft Drinks (12 oz.)	
Sugar-Free Mr. PIBB	58.8
Mountain Dew	54.0
Mello Yello	52.8
TAB	46.8
Coca-Cola	45.6
Diet Coke	45.6
Shasta Cola	44.4
Shasta Cherry Cola	44.4
Shasta Diet Cola	44.4
Mr. PIBB	40.8
Dr. Pepper	39.6
Sugar-Free Dr. Pepper	39.6
Big Red	38.4
Sugar-Free Big Red	38.4
Pepsi-Cola	38.4
Aspen	36.0
Diet Pepsi	36.0
Pepsi Light	36.0
RC Cola	36.0
Diet Rite	36.0
Kick	31.2
Canada Dry Jamaica Cola	30.0
Canada Dry Diet Cola	1.2
Cocoa and Chocolate	
Cocoa beverage (5 oz.)	4
Chocolate milk beverage (8 oz.)	5
Milk chocolate (1 oz.)	6
Dark chocolate, semi-sweet (1 oz.)	20
Baker's chocolate (1 oz.)	26
Chocolate-flavored syrup (1 oz.)	4
Nonprescription Drugs	
Weight-Control Aids	
Dex-A-Diet II	200
Dexatrim	200
Dexatrim Extra Strength	200
Dietac capsules	200
Maximum Strength Appedrine	100
Prolamine	140
Alertness Tablets	
Nodoz	100
Vivarin	200
Analgesic/Pain Relief	
Anacin	32
Maximum Strength Anacin	32
Excedrin	65
Midol	32
Vanquish	33
Diuretics	
Aqua-Ban	100
Maximum Strength Aqua-Ban Plus	200
Permathene H2 Off	200
Cold/Allergy Remedies	
Coryban-D capsules	30
Triaminicin tablets	30
Dristan Decongestant tablets	16
Dristan A-F Decongestant tablets	16
Duradyne-Forte	30

symptoms disappear in their babies. Other common offenders are citrus fruits, eggs, wheat, fish, pork, and nuts.

ATTAINING AND MAINTAINING A HEALTHY WEIGHT

Many women have been misled into believing that by six weeks postpartum they will have returned to their prepregnant weights and sizes, and will be able to resume their previous activity levels. After all, the baby has been born, so extra pounds should be shed relatively easily, shouldn't they? However hopeful this notion may be, it is not realistic. Regaining your figure may take considerably more time and effort than anticipated.

Limiting Weight Loss

The extra body weight that was needed to support pregnancy will be shed rather quickly. After several weeks, your weight may level off. At this time, you will probably weigh five to fifteen pounds more than you did when you conceived. The remaining fat stored in your body will provide extra energy to fuel the production of breast milk during your baby's first four months. As you nurse, the fat stores will be slowly depleted, making weight loss almost effortless. However, if you lose weight too rapidly by limiting your intake of calories, you may be unable to make enough milk to satisfy your baby. In addition, rapid weight loss can release those contaminants that are stored in body fat, exposing your baby to large amounts of toxic substances. Slow, steady weight loss will be safest for you and your baby.

Regaining Body Tone

While trying to regain your figure, another fact you should take into consideration is that during pregnancy your pelvic bones were spread apart and your abdominal tissues were stretched. It may take as long as nine months for the bones to return to their former positions and the muscles to regain their tone. If you wore a size 10 before pregnancy, you may have to wear a size 12 after delivery—and this may be true even after those extra pounds have disappeared. Only exercise and time will get you back into shape. Further dieting is not the answer, so don't starve yourself in an attempt to flatten your tummy! An exercise program for postpartum women will help you attain your goals.

Cutting Calories

If you do attempt to lose weight while nursing, you can safely reduce your calories by modifying the guidelines provided in the Pregnant/ Lactating column of Table 2.1 on page 25. Reduce your consumption of eggs to one per day. In addition, fat and sugar consumption should be decreased by drinking skim milk rather than whole, choosing unflavored yogurt and lowfat cottage cheese, and omitting pudding and ice cream. These alterations will provide approximately 200 less calories per day, enabling you to lose about three pounds per month. If psychological factors cause you to eat, try substituting another activity, or at least choose low-calorie, nutritious foods. Gradual weight loss is best for your health, is most likely to result in permanent weight loss, and, perhaps most important, will ensure your ability to produce enough milk for your baby.

Once your baby starts eating solid foods, you will need to cut down on your own food intake in order to prevent weight gain. This is the time when many women fail to lose weight, or even put on a few pounds. They have grown used to eating a certain amount of food and find it difficult to eat less. Gradually cutting out snacks and reducing the portion sizes as your baby nurses less will help you to avoid weight gain. Just realizing that a potential problem exists may motivate you to limit your intake.

Avoiding Fad Diets

One thing you must avoid is a fad-type diet that emphasizes one food group while eliminating others. Many of these diets are unhealthy, resulting in undernutrition and a tired, worn-out feeling. There are no magical methods of weight loss. Eating less and exercising more are the only reliable paths to permanent weight loss. Natural food diets and vegetarian diets, however, can be very nutritious when food selection is done carefully. Before going on such a diet, you should become familiar with ways of combining proteins and learn about the nutrients contained in each food you wish to include. Be aware that vegetarians need to consciously choose foods that are rich in iron and the B vitamins—especially Vitamin B12—in order to prevent deficiencies.

While pregnancy stimulates a nutritional awakening in many women, lactation continues the learning period, providing further opportunities to gain new knowledge about dietary practices. Although it may initially require extra time and thought to modify your eating habits, your efforts to improve your diet will not only produce immediate benefits for you and your baby, but may be the start of a lifetime of good nutrition for your entire family.

AT A GLANCE

Eating Well for You and Your Baby

Recommendations for Improving Your Diet

- Eat a balanced diet with 3 meals and 2 to 3 nutritious snacks a day.
- Improve your diet gradually, cutting out those practices that you believe are most harmful.
- Cut food costs by planning meals, purchasing sale items, using a shopping list, and substituting less expensive sources of protein for meat.
- Eat a variety of foods, making sure that your diet contains foods from all four of the basic food groups—milk, meats, fruits and vegetables, and grains.

Special Diet Suggestions While Breastfeeding

- Consume approximately 2,200 calories per day.
- Drink to satisfy your thirst—6 to 8 cups of liquid is adequate.
- Every day, eat foods that are rich in calcium.
- Avoid foods that seem to give your baby indigestion.
- Limit caffeine if your baby is unusually wakeful or fussy.
- Avoid potential allergens if your baby shows signs of allergies.

Postpartum Weight Control

- Expect to lose weight rapidly for the first few weeks postpartum, and then to have your weight level off.
- After the first few weeks, lose weight gradually to maintain your milk supply.
- To lose weight, cut out about 200 calories per day, eliminating milk products with high fat and sugar contents.
- Avoid fad diets.
- As your baby begins eating solid foods and nursing less, prevent weight gain by cutting down your own food intake.

6
Getting Off to the Best Possible Start

Like any new experience, the first few nursings may be scary or make you feel awkward or anxious. You will want to do everything just right, and yet will be unsure how to go about it. Take heart. You have a companion in this adventure; your baby needs to learn about nursing too! Together, the two of you will experiment as you find comfortable positions for breastfeeding, learn how to go about the mechanics of feeding, and enjoy the rewards of a close, warm relationship.

The first few days after birth, nursings will probably take place in a hospital setting. Breastfeeding in the hospital is easier than nursing at home in some respects and more difficult in others. In the hospital, you will be free from household responsibilities and will be able to concentrate totally on your baby. You also will have a staff of nurses to assist you with feedings and instruct you in infant care. In the privacy of your own home, however, you will be able to relax and enjoy the company of your family. You can nurse your baby whenever he is hungry, without regard to hospital rules and schedules. You will be able to establish a routine without interference from a myriad of hospital employees, ranging from maintenance to food service personnel. Since some of your breastfeeding practices will differ from hospital to home, the material in each discussion within this chapter will address both situations. Advice on breastfeeding in the hospital will be presented first, followed by adaptations for nursing at home, when applicable.

PREPARING FOR THE FIRST NURSINGS

Especially at the beginning of your breastfeeding experience, you will need to plan ahead for nursings so that you can feed your baby without delay when he is hungry. Before your baby becomes hungry, take care of your own needs, collect all the items you may require, and arrange your bed or chair for nursing. These preparations will make feedings more enjoyable for both of you, eliminating the need to get up in the middle of a feeding or to sit through a feeding feeling uncomfortable. Taking the time before feedings to settle your baby down or to rouse him to wakefulness, as necessary, will result in more satisfactory nursings.

Establishing a feeding routine will help make nursings go smoothly, teach your baby what to expect, and condition your baby to respond to your cues. The following discussion offers suggestions for nursing that you may wish to adapt to suit your lifestyle and needs. The basic steps presented will help you to prepare for the early feedings, and will probably become second nature as you continue to nurse your baby. Each of the listed steps is discussed in detail on the pages that follow.

Steps in Your Nursing Routine:

1. Prepare yourself and your baby for the nursing.
   - Take care of your personal needs.
   - Rouse or calm your baby, as necessary.
   - Relax and establish letdown.
2. Select a comfortable nursing position.
3. Establish a sound feeding routine.
   - Put your baby on the breast.
   - Nurse on one breast until your baby releases the nipple.

- Nurse on the second breast if your baby is willing.
- Base the frequency of feedings on your baby's needs.

4. End the feeding.
   - Let your baby release the nipple.
   - Burp your baby.
   - Properly care for your breasts.

Prepare Yourself for Each Nursing

To prepare for each nursing, first take care of your personal needs. Use the toilet; wash your hands; fluff your pillows; and gather reading materials, a beverage, burp cloth, and whatever else you may want to have with you. Try to begin these preparations about ten minutes before the planned feeding time or, if rooming-in, before your baby fusses too much from hunger. There is no need to wash your breasts before each feeding, since the natural oils on your nipples act to discourage bacterial growth. Soaps and alcohol pads can dry and irritate the skin, as well as create an unappetizing taste for your baby. While there is no harm in wiping your nipples with clear water, this is usually only necessary when milk residue is present.

Prepare Your Baby for Each Nursing

In order to nurse successfully, your baby should be hungry enough to be interested in the breast, but not so hungry that he fusses or cries loudly. If your baby is in the nursery on demand feedings, either ask the staff to bring him to you before he gets too fussy or check on him every couple of hours yourself. If you are restricted to scheduled feedings, you may not be able to nurse at the best time, and may have to wake or calm your baby for nursings. If your baby stays with you in your hospital room, you will be able to nurse him whenever he is hungry. Similarly, when you are at home, you will be able to watch and listen for him to awaken, and feed him when he begins to show signs of hunger such as avid sucking on his thumb or fingers, alertness with a lot of movement, or a succession of short cries.

Depending on your hospital's procedures, you may need to consider diaper changes in conjunction with feeding times. When your baby is hungry and you must change his diaper, it is usually best to nurse him on one breast, change his diaper, and then nurse him on the second breast. This practice, in fact, works well in a number of cases. For example, a fussy baby will be satisfied and calmed by immediate nursing, while a sleepy baby will be encouraged to stay awake by a mid-feeding diaper change. Diapering before feedings often works well when the baby is quietly alert and does not tend to fall asleep in the middle of feedings. Pre-feeding diaper changes can also be used if your baby is not very hungry when he is brought into your room. In this instance, you can take the time to hold him, talk to him, and change his diaper before nursing him. In the early weeks, diaper changes after feedings are not usually recommended. Many newborn babies do not like to be disturbed after nursing, preferring instead to fall asleep. Regardless of your routine, arrange for lengthy feeding times—at least forty-five minutes—to allow for preparation, interaction, and nursing.

When Your Baby Is Sleepy

During the first few days after birth, your baby may be so sleepy from the delivery that he will be unable to stay awake for feedings. Because newborn babies sleep most of the time, you may need to wake your baby so that he will nurse often enough to establish a good milk supply. Conditioning your baby to the same routine before every feeding will help him to become accustomed to nursing. You can also massage your breasts and hand express some milk before feedings in order to encourage letdown so that your baby will not tire quickly from vigorous suckling. Short, frequent feedings, too, will reduce the possibility of his falling asleep during the feeding. If your breasts are still full after a feeding, empty them manually or ask the hospital personnel for a breast pump. When you are home, you will be able to save your milk and offer it to your baby with a bottle or eyedropper at another time. In the early weeks, supplemental feedings and bottles of water should be avoided whenever possible so that your baby will spend his alert times at the breast.

If your baby is sleepy, you may have difficulty rousing him for feedings. The following techniques will help you to awaken your baby enough to interest him in nursing.

- Pick your baby up and loosen or remove his blankets to expose him to the air.
- Change your baby's diaper.
- Unclothe your baby and swab him with lukewarm water, or immerse him in bath water.
- Hold your baby in a sitting or standing position and gently move his arms back and forth.
- Stimulate your baby's sense of smell by bringing him close to your breast.
- Express some breast milk onto your baby's lips to stimulate his sense of taste.
- Rub your nipple against the baby's cheek to stimulate his rooting reflex (see page 80 for information on the rooting reflex).
- Once the nipple is in your baby's mouth, gently stroke his neck from the chin back to encourage suckling.
- Talk softly to your baby and try to maintain eye contact with him.

When Your Baby Is Fussy

It can be very frustrating to try to nurse your baby when he is fussy. Since he cannot cry and nurse at the same time, try to nurse him before he becomes so agitated that he cannot be calmed easily. If your baby's cries are not quieted when he is offered the breast, you will need to determine if his cries are being caused by something other than hunger. Could he be overheated from too much clothing or bedding? Is he chilled from a wet diaper or insufficient clothing? Is the texture of the material next to his body rough and irritating? Is his stomach overly full because of a gas bubble that needs to be brought up? Might the sights, sounds, and smells around him be upsetting? In addition to correcting these possible causes of discomfort, you may wish to try the following:

- Handle your baby in a manner that is slow, calm, deliberate, and firm.
- Cuddle, hold, walk, talk, and sing softly to your baby.
- Swaddle your baby firmly in his blanket to restrict movements that may startle him.
- Stimulate your baby's rooting reflex to signal the beginning of a feeding.
- Provide constant rhythmic movements by rocking your baby.
- Later, when you return home, a car ride, a swing, or walking may also help.
- Provide constant soothing sounds by humming, talking, or turning on the television. At home, try music or the sounds of a vacuum cleaner or dishwasher.
- If your baby seems overstimulated, draw the curtains, turn off the lights and television, and nurse in a dark, quiet room.
- Use short, frequent feedings and burp your baby often.
- Massage your baby's body slowly and firmly.
- Let your baby suck on your index finger.
- Change your diet, removing allergens that can be passed to your baby through your milk.
- At home, increase body and skin contact by sleeping and bathing with your baby and carrying him in a baby sling against your chest.
- At home, remove allergens from your baby's environment—dust, pets, wool blankets and clothing, fumes, and cigarette smoke.

Relax and Establish Letdown

Once you are positioned with your baby and ready to nurse, take a few minutes to relax together. Talk to your baby while arranging pillows and getting comfortable. A few deep breaths and several moments of quiet reflection will help your milk to let down. A gentle massage of your baby and your breasts, too, will help to eliminate tension while conditioning the letdown reflex.

If you have difficulty relaxing, try removing all potential disturbances—take the phone off the hook, put a "Do Not Disturb" sign on your door, and play some relaxing music. A healthy, positive attitude about breastfeeding, thoughts about all the ways in which nursing will benefit your baby, and an enjoyment of the closeness you're sharing with him will help you to approach nursing with confidence.

Letdown usually takes place very shortly after your baby begins nursing, and occurs a number of times during each feeding. While the letdown reflex is often unpredictable during the first few days—or even weeks—you will know that it is working if you observe any of the signs listed in Table 6.1. However, it is possible that there will be no obvious signs of letdown. The only indication that it is taking place may be your baby's satisfaction and well-being.

Table 6.1 Signs of Letdown

In Mother	In Baby
• Strong uterine contractions. • Sudden fullness or tightness in the breasts. • A tingling sensation. • A shooting pain. • Relief of pressure from the breasts.	• A change in his sucking pattern—gulping, gagging, and more pronounced swallowing. • Pulling away from the breast due to excess milk flow. • Leaking of milk from the breasts. • 6 to 8 wet diapers a day with no supplemental fluids. • Satisfaction at the end of each nursing.

POSITIONING YOUR BABY

The single most important aspect of breastfeeding management is the technique of positioning your baby on your breast. Positioning can determine how much milk your baby gets, how your baby sucks, whether or not your nipples become sore, how much milk you produce, how long your baby nurses at each feeding, and whether breastfeeding is successful.

One of the best ways to tell if your baby is well positioned is to assess your comfort level. In a good position, you should be relaxed, with all parts of your body well supported. While your baby is nursing, your breasts should not be under stress, and you should not feel pain. Your baby also will be relaxed when well positioned, with all of his body well supported, his mouth aligned slightly below the center of your breast, and his body turned tummy-to-tummy to you.

Selecting a Nursing Position

When selecting a nursing position, you will want to consider your own comfort and your baby's abilities. For most nursings, many women are happy using the cradle (also called Madonna) position, with the baby lying across the mother's abdomen. There are a variety of other nursing positions for both sitting up and lying down. You can experiment to find the ones that are most comfortable for you and your baby. Before each nursing, give thought to which position you will use and how you will hold your baby. This will determine whether you should prepare a chair or bed for nursing, and which pillows you will need to make yourself comfortable. (Pillows make a great shower gift for a pregnant or new mother!) Also consider placing a small pillow or folded blanket under your baby to raise him up to the breast, so that he does not pull on the tissue during nursing.

The Cradle Nursing Position

To nurse in the cradle position, sit in a comfortable chair or raised hospital bed. Make certain that you have adequate sup-

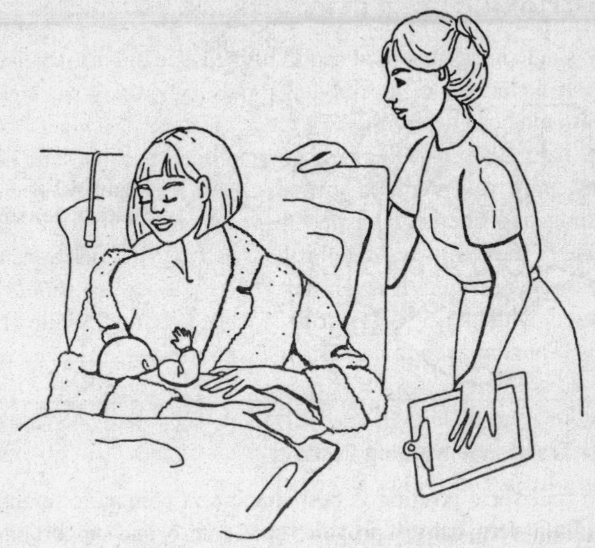

Figure 6.1 Cradle Nursing Position

port for your arms, back, and legs. As shown in Figure 6.1, place your baby across your lap, positioning him so that he is held tummy-to-tummy to you. Use pillows to raise him to the level of your breasts. If no pillows are available, raise his head by crossing one of your legs over the other. If you are nursing from the right breast, support your baby's head and back with your right arm and use your left hand to guide your breast into his mouth. Make sure that his head, trunk, and legs follow a straight line from his neck to his navel.

The Football Nursing Position

The football nursing position is a sitting position that can be helpful if your baby prefers lying on a particular side. Referring to Figure 6.2, place your baby on his side on pillows along your body, with his feet back behind your arm. Support your breast with the opposite hand. While cradling his head and back with the arm nearest his head, guide him toward your breast.

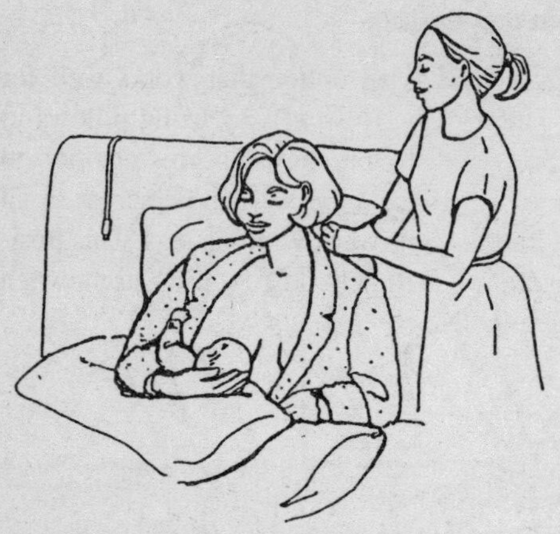

Figure 6.2
Football Nursing Position

The Transverse Nursing Position

The transverse position is best suited to a premature infant or small full-term baby. It provides good control and support of the baby's head and body. This position is similar to the cradle position in that the baby lies across your abdomen. However, in the transverse position, the baby's head and body are held by your left arm when the baby nurses on your right breast, as depicted in Figure 6.3.

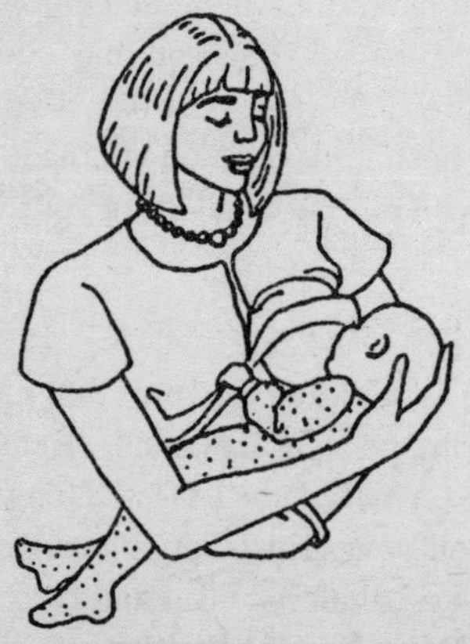

Figure 6.3
Transverse Nursing Position

The Tailor-Style Nursing Position

Sitting tailor or Indian style is an option that works well for nursing an older or larger baby. However, by using pillows to raise your baby to breast level, you can adapt this position to meet the needs of your newborn. A toddler can lie across or sit on your lap, or can straddle your waist with his legs. This position, as shown in Figure 6.4, will help prevent back strain when no back support is available.

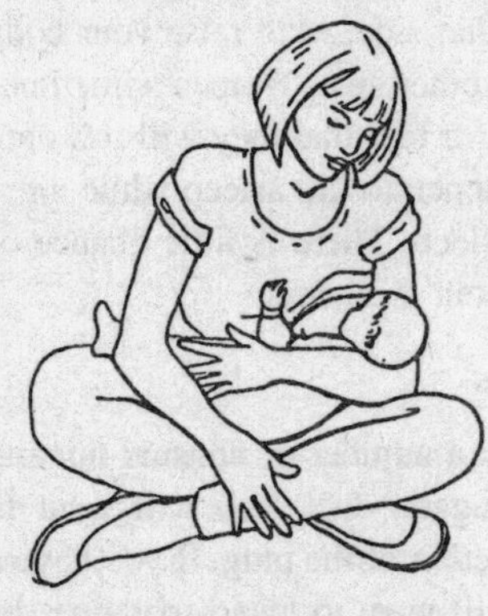

Figure 6.4 Tailor-Style Nursing Position

Nursing While Lying Down

Nursing while lying down can be very relaxing and enjoyable. While this position may be awkward at first, you may come to prefer it, as it will allow you to catch up on your rest. The easiest way to nurse in a reclining position is to lie on your side with your knees bent slightly and with pillows supporting your head, back, and upper leg.

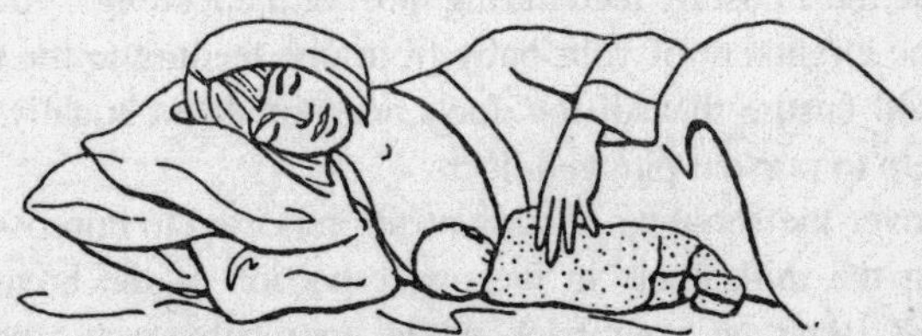

Figure 6.5 Lying-Down Nursing Position

Place your baby on his side next to you on a pillow or blanket, raising him to the level of your lower breast. You can either place your lower arm under your head and use your upper arm to draw your baby close, or place your lower arm around your baby's head and back. Figure 6.5 depicts one way of nursing in this position.

To offer the opposite breast, simply roll toward your baby and rearrange the bedding to provide proper support. Other ways to offer the opposite breast are to hold your baby close to your chest and roll him over to the other side, or to raise your body over your baby and move to his other side. Women sometimes avoid nursing while lying down for fear that they will roll onto the baby in their sleep. If you happen to fall asleep while nursing, it will probably be a light sleep. There is little chance of your rolling onto your baby without awakening.

Less Common Nursing Positions

Mothers have been known to try a number of unusual nursing positions. When you have a plugged duct, you will want to place your baby's jaw in the direction of the plug. If you have a sore spot on your nipple, you will want to avoid irritating the area. There is even a position to control the strong flow of milk.

When the milk flows too quickly from your breast, you can position your baby so that the milk flow is slowed. Called posture feeding, this method requires that you lie on your back with pillows supporting your head and shoulders. You can place your baby either on top of your torso or alongside of you on pillows, supporting his forehead with the heel of your hand. If you find that you must posture feed during most of the feedings, you can vary the alignment of your baby from one feeding to the next. This will ensure that all the ducts are stimulated equally, and will help to prevent plugged ducts.

The over-the-shoulder nursing position is used to improve the flow in the milk ducts in the upper portion of the breast. It involves lying on your back while your baby rests, tummy

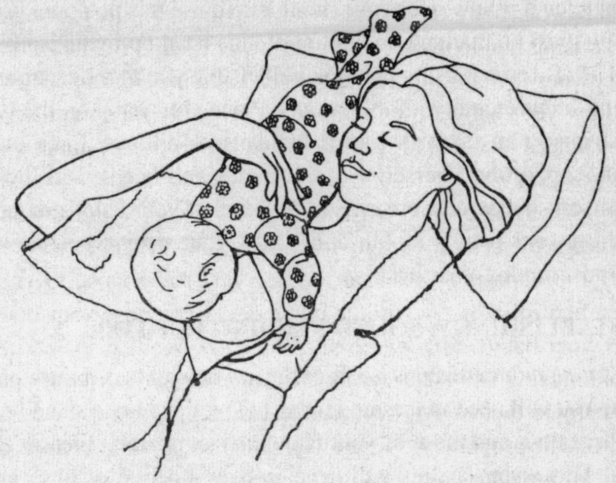

Figure 6.6 Over-the-Shoulder Nursing Position

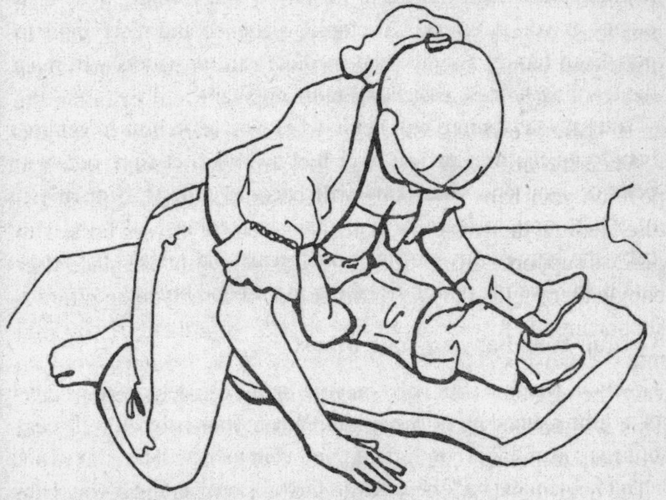

Figure 6.7 All-Fours Nursing Position

down, on a pillow over your shoulder. To use this position, your baby must be mature enough to hold his head up by himself.

The all-fours nursing position will enable you to move around your baby to empty all milk ducts. Place your baby on the bed and raise him up with folded blankets or pillows. Lean over him, supporting yourself on your hands and knees, and lower yourself so that your breast is at the level of your baby's mouth. Adjust your baby's mouth and adjust your baby's position to avoid straining your back.

ESTABLISHING A SOUND FEEDING ROUTINE

Learning to breastfeed is a part of the newness of becoming a parent. You will need to master new techniques and understand how your actions and those of your baby interact to affect breastfeeding. This understanding will develop over a period of time, and will depend on the intimate contact and communication between you and your baby. You will become partners in a new experience, learning from each other and acquiring and refining your techniques as you progress. Developing patience and receiving support from family, friends, and medical care providers will make the learning process easier and more enjoyable.

Your new adventure will begin when you learn how to get your baby onto the breast. You may feel awkward at first; but, with practice, you and your baby will become experts. Similarly, it may take time to learn how to manage feedings, allowing your baby the opportunity to finish one breast and release the nipple and then have the option of taking the second breast.

Getting Your Baby on Your Breast

How you position your baby on your breast can determine whether or not breastfeeding is successful. When your baby is well positioned, you will feel comfortable, and your baby will be relaxed and able to obtain the milk he needs to thrive. Determining if your baby is well positioned is easier once you understand how the breast is drawn into your baby's mouth and what happens during sucking.

Sucking involves the baby's entire mouth—his lips, gums, tongue, cheeks, and hard and soft palates. First, he uses his tongue to draw the nipple far back into his mouth and mold the areola into a coneshaped extension of the nipple. Then, while suction holds the breast in his mouth, his tongue ripples backwards and his gums move up and down to press the milk out of the collecting sinuses beneath the areola. It is thus very important for your baby to take a good part of the areola, as well as the nipple, into his mouth.

Establishing an effective feeding routine will condition your baby to properly grasp the breast at the beginning of every nursing (see Figure 6.8). Lay your baby on his side, and hold him close to you so that his mouth is aligned slightly below the center of your nipple. Make sure that your arm is supported so that it is not bearing his weight. Cup your free hand to form the letter "C," with your thumb on top and your fingers curved below. Place this hand around your breast. This method of breast support is called the C-hold. Brush your nipple against his bottom lip, and your baby should automatically respond with the **rooting reflex** by opening his mouth wide. Guide your breast far back into your baby's mouth. You will know that your baby is positioned on the breast correctly if both his nose and chin are touching the breast, and his lips are flanged outward around the breast (like the mouth of a fish). If you gently pull down his bottom lip, you should be able to see that his tongue is cupped and lying over his lower gum.

Because your baby's mouth will be open for only a short time, you may not be able to position your breast correctly the first time. Instead of trying to push your breast in farther or attempting to manipulate your baby's head, it is best to remove your breast, relax, and begin again. Take a deep breath and laugh it off; these first attempts can be very humorous. Bring your baby close to you, brush your nipple against his mouth, and try again.

If your baby seems uninterested in your breast, entice him by expressing a few drops of milk onto his lips. When encouraging

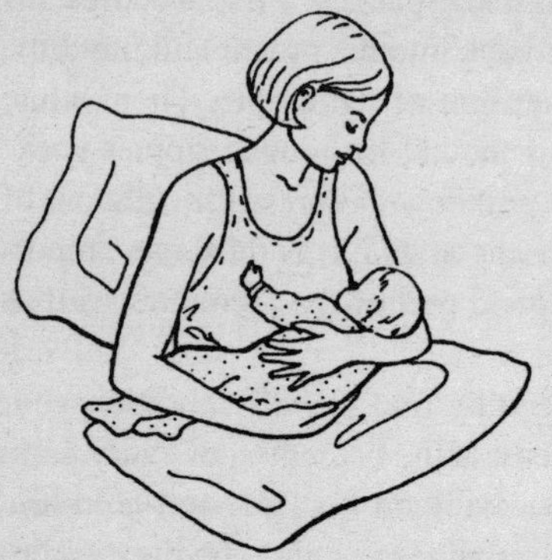

1. Support your arms and back to avoid strain. Bring your baby close to you with his body facing yours.

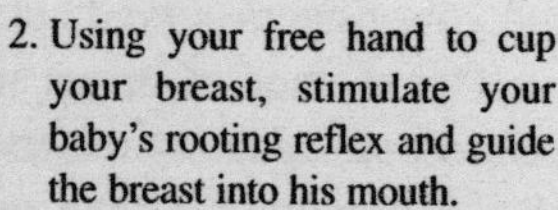

2. Using your free hand to cup your breast, stimulate your baby's rooting reflex and guide the breast into his mouth.

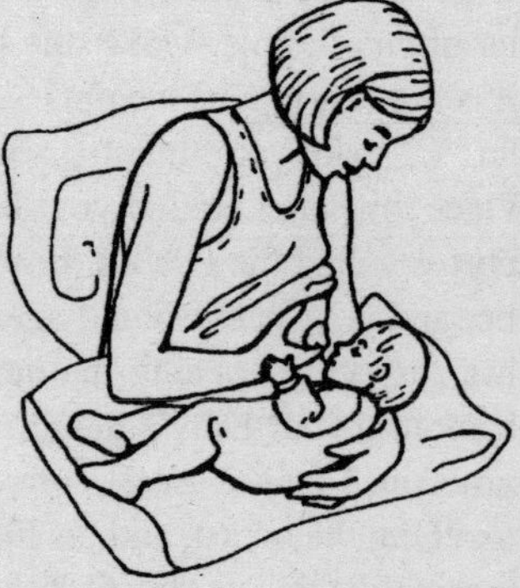

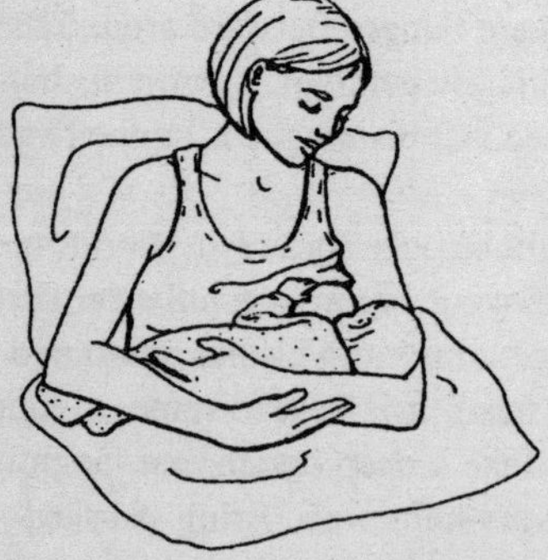

3. With the breast well into your baby's mouth, continue holding him closely throughout the feeding.

Figure 6.8 Sequence for Getting Your Baby Onto Your Breast

your baby to take your breast, be careful not to touch his opposite cheek with your hand. His rooting reflex will cause him to turn toward the touch and away from your breast. After several tries, you should be able to start breastfeeding.

If your breast slips out of your baby's mouth, adjust your baby's position so the breast lies naturally in his mouth, with your nipple aligned slightly below center and close enough so that your baby's chin and nose both touch the breast. There is no need to hold the breast away from your baby's nose. He will be able to breathe through the space that lies between his nose and mouth. If your breasts are large or if your baby has difficulty keeping the breast in his mouth, you may wish to use the C-hold to support the breast with the palm of your hand during the entire feeding.

Providing Sufficient Stimulation for Milk Production

When your baby nurses, his sucking will be most vigorous and rapid at the beginning of the feeding. As letdown of the milk occurs, the sucking rate will slow down, and your baby will suck and swallow rhythmically. When the flow of milk decreases, your baby will suck more rapidly again until the flow increases. The initial milk, or foremilk, contains less fat and more water than the later hindmilk. As the milk flows through the ducts, it will dislodge the fat particles from the duct walls, and these particles will accumulate in the milk as the feeding progresses. When the flow of milk becomes very slow, your baby will gently release the breast from his mouth.

In order to continue the feeding, you can offer the other breast. If your baby is still hungry, he will accept the second breast and nurse until the milk flow has diminished, and then release the second breast to signal the end of the feeding. Or, he may nurse only a short time on the second breast before ending the feeding. If your baby is satisfied by the feeding on the first breast, he may not want to nurse on the second breast at all. How long your baby nurses on the second breast is not of great importance. However, it is crucial that he nurse long enough on the first breast to receive a significant amount of high-fat milk, and to remove enough milk to signal your body to continue making milk at the present rate.

If your baby nurses on only one breast at each feeding, he may have fewer problems with indigestion and spitting up because he is not taking in more milk than he can handle at one time. Also, your baby may want to nurse more often if he is nursing primarily on one breast per feeding. However, his weight gain may be greater than it would if you were nursing him for a limited time on both breasts at each feeding, because he is receiving more calories from the high-fat hindmilk.

If the less-nursed breast begins to feel full before the next feeding, express milk for comfort. To ensure that your breasts receive equal stimulation, alternate the breast with which you start each feeding. If you started with the left breast at the last feeding, start with the right breast at the next feeding. To help yourself remember which side to use each time, you may wish to try one of the suggestions listed below:

- Leave your bra flap down on the second side, ready for the next feeding.
- Fasten a safety pin to the second side of your bra.
- Move your watch to the wrist on the second side.
- Lay your baby down with his head at the end of the crib that corresponds to the second breast as you face the side of the crib.

In order to ensure that your baby gains an adequate amount of weight, the technique of **Alternate Breast Massage** can be used during feedings.[1] Mothers who use this method experience less engorgement and nipple soreness, while their babies tend to retain their interest in nursing longer.[2] To utilize this technique, first observe your baby's manner of sucking. You will notice that your baby's sucking will be most vigorous and rapid at the beginning of the feeding. After letdown occurs, his sucking pattern will become long and slow as he rhythmically compresses the collecting sinuses with his gums. As less milk becomes available, the pattern will again become rapid and shallow, with alternating periods of rest and bursts of nursing. As soon as you notice that the nursing pattern has grown rapid and shallow, begin massaging your breast. Starting under your arm, gently stroke the breast from the chest wall to your nipple several times. Although your baby will stop sucking during the massage, he will take several long sucks each time you stop, removing the milk that you just brought down from the alveoli. As you feel your breast soften beneath your fingers, move your hand to a new position and continue to alternate the massage with your baby's sucking until your entire breast has been softened. Remember to use the massage only after your baby's sucking pattern has changed to shallow bursts. Massaging too early in the feeding can result in a rapid flow of milk that your baby may be unable to handle.

Knowing How Often and How Long to Nurse

While learning to manage nursings, keep in mind that two very important aspects of successful breastfeeding are duration and frequency. For the most part, your baby will establish the length and time of each feeding session. However, you always have the option of increasing or decreasing nursing times and adjusting the time between feedings in order to improve breastfeeding or adapt it to your lifestyle. For instance, nipple pain may be relieved by a change in nursing schedule. Nursing times can be altered to be more compatible with household or employment responsibilities. Improving the nursing schedule can also ensure that your breasts receive enough stimulation to meet your baby's nutritional needs.

The Duration of Feedings

In the past, nursing times were limited because it was believed that longer periods at the breast contributed to nipple soreness. There is no evidence to show that unlimited sucking in any way contributes to the development of sore nipples. In fact, research shows that unlimited sucking time actually results in more successful breastfeeding. While 80 to 90 percent of the milk volume is obtained during the first four minutes at each breast, most of the calories are present in the fatty hindmilk, which is obtained later in the feeding. To ensure the well-being of your baby therefore, fairly long nursing times are recommended, especially during the first few weeks.

Some hospitals still recommend that early feedings be limited to five to seven minutes per breast. However, this does not take into consideration the slower initial letdown times or the need for adequate stimulation for milk production. The duration of these early feedings should be dictated by your baby's interest and by the speed with which he removes milk. You can determine how long to nurse by watching your baby's sucking pattern. Initial sucking comes in quick bursts that stimulate letdown. When more milk flows, slower rhythmical sucking occurs. As the milk flow subsides, your baby will again suck in quicker bursts, until another letdown occurs. When the flow has decreased to a very slow rate and further bursts of sucking do not increase the flow, your baby will release the breast from his mouth. This is a good time to try burping your baby. Then you can offer him the second breast, repeating the nursing pattern that occurred on the first breast if he is interested in nursing longer. Be aware that a newborn is often very sleepy, and may alternately suck and rest while keeping the breast in his mouth. This does not necessarily indicate that he is ready to end the feeding, but especially long resting periods may mean that your baby is finished.

As your baby matures, he will become more efficient at removing milk. Your baby may then need considerably less time to obtain most of the milk in your breasts. Since you are continuously producing milk, your breasts will never be totally empty, although only a few drops may be available after long nursing sessions. Be aware, though, that your baby may continue to nurse even after the available milk has been removed from both breasts. Babies usually require this non-nutritive nursing to fulfill their sucking needs.

The Frequency of Feedings

For successful breastfeeding, the frequency of feedings should vary according to your baby's needs. At least nine feedings per day are essential soon after birth to build your milk supply and to prevent an accumulation of your baby's body waste products, which can result in jaundice. Most newborns nurse at irregular intervals that are one and a half to three hours apart—or ten to twelve times in each twenty-four hour period. During the first week, it will be best not to let your baby go more than three hours from the beginning of one feeding to the beginning of the next.

After about six weeks, a pattern will probably develop in which your baby nurses every two to three hours, with one longer stretch at night. Some babies, however, sleep longer during the day; to modify their schedules, you will have to awaken them for feedings. During the first week, you can expect one to three feedings per night. This schedule will help bring your milk in sooner and will build up your supply more quickly. Be sure to advise hospital personnel that you wish to nurse during the night. The practice of nursery personnel's giving your baby formula so you can sleep is harmful rather than helpful, as it interferes with milk production.

Some hospital schedules give you access to your baby only at certain times. This can get you off to a slow start by limiting nursings to less than nine a day. One way to increase nursings is to feed your baby twice during each visit—once at the beginning of the visit and once at the end. Another possible alternative is to obtain permission to feed your baby in the nursery between scheduled visits. Often, you can switch over to rooming-in midway through your stay. If none of these options is available to you, let your baby's doctor know that you would like him to leave orders in the nursery allowing you to nurse every two or three hours, or on the basis of need. When you return home, you will be able to nurse as often as desired.

ENDING THE FEEDING

Just as the way in which you begin the feeding is important to successful breastfeeding, the way in which you end the feeding will contribute to a more enjoyable nursing experience. By guiding your baby off the breast without stressing the tissue, and by properly caring for your breasts after each feeding, you will help to prevent sore nipples. Burping your baby during and after nursings will make him more comfortable and reduce the possibility of his spitting up. As you gain experience, these techniques will probably become second nature to you, and you may wonder that you were ever unsure of how to manage them.

Guiding Your Baby Off the Breast

As the flow of milk subsides at the breast, your baby's sucking pattern will change to alternating periods of rest and bursts of nursing. In most cases, he will then release the breast spontaneously. Or, he may become drowsy, suck more slowly, open his jaw, or begin "chewing" his way off the nipple. If "chewing" occurs, you will need to remove the breast from your baby's mouth to prevent damage to the tissue. Note that this may be a sign that your baby is not positioned well back on the breast, and is not able to remove the milk easily. To remove your baby from the breast, break the suction by inserting your finger into the corner of his mouth between his gums. If your baby consistently clamps his gums together to retain the breast at the end of the feeding, try to anticipate his actions and insert your finger between his gums ahead of time to avoid tissue damage.

Burping Your Baby

Like bottle-fed babies, breast-fed babies need to be burped regularly, as they can still gulp air while suckling. You can reduce the amount of air swallowed by feeding your baby frequently, so that his hunger does not cause him to begin the feeding by sucking frantically. Because a forceful letdown can also cause your baby to gulp and swallow air, you may wish to express milk before beginning the feeding so that your baby can nurse calmly. If your baby has been crying hard, he may need to be burped before a feeding to expel any air that he may have already swallowed. Burping will make your baby more comfortable, decrease gas pains, and lessen the chance of his spitting up. It is a good idea to burp your baby after he nurses on each breast, and, after the feeding, to wait as long as twenty minutes for the last bubble

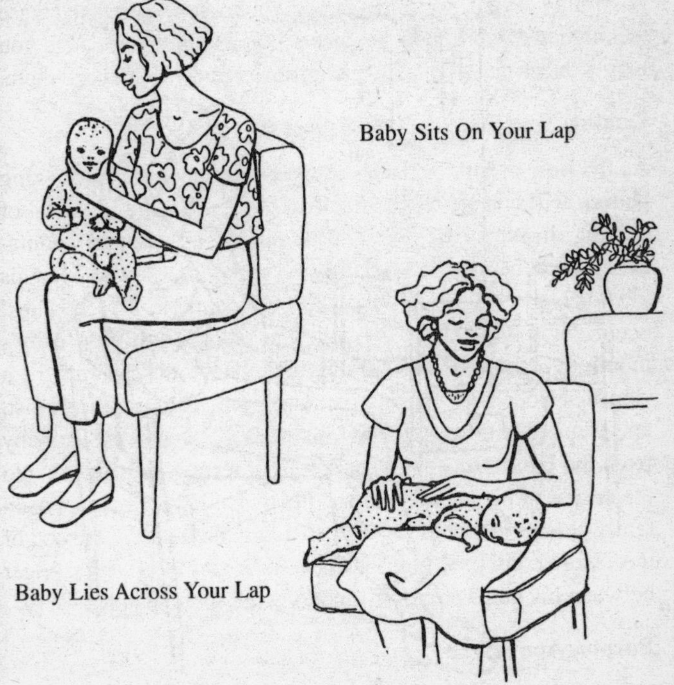

Figure 6.9 Common Burping Positions

to come up. This will be a good time for you to get to know your baby as you hold him and talk to him.

You can burp your baby while he is sitting on your lap, lying on his stomach across your lap, or lying against your shoulder (see Figure 6.9). Gently rub his back in a circular motion or pat him with firm pressure, starting at the bottom of his back and working upward. Sometimes the excess air will come up readily. More often, though, it will take some time, and you may have to experiment to discover which method of burping works best for your baby. Fathers are often successful in creating unique and amazingly effective burping positions.

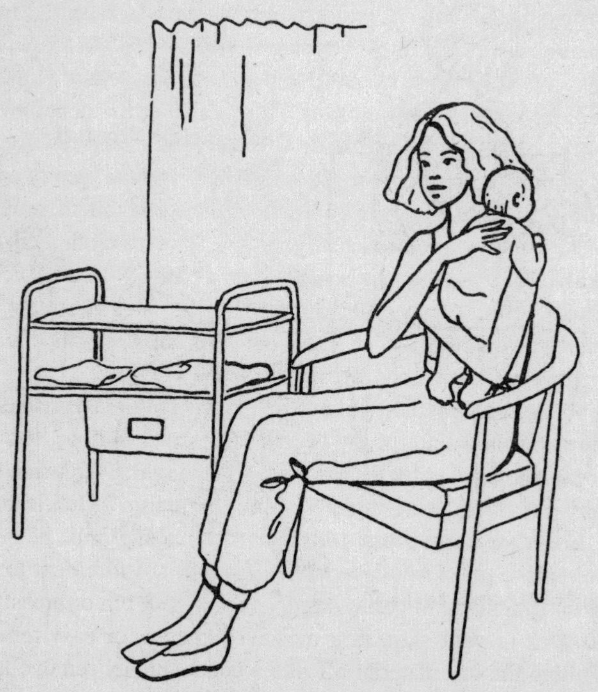

Baby Lies Against Your Shoulder

Occasionally, your baby may not burp within a reasonable time after a feeding. You can lay him on his stomach in his crib so that the warmth and pressure of his bed can help the bubble of air to rise. Another way to burp your baby—and to reduce spitting up—is to lay him on his right side. Place rolled blankets in front and back of him to ensure that he will not roll over. As the stomach opens to the esophagus on the left side, your baby will be less likely to bring up milk when he lies in this position. An older baby who is alert may be placed in an infant seat or swing until the bubble of air is expelled.

Caring for Your Breasts

Proper breast care at the end of a feeding is essential to the maintenance of healthy breast and nipple skin. While you are burping your baby, leave your bra flaps down, allowing your nipples to dry. Excess moisture creates an environment in which bacteria can grow, and milk is a very rich medium for this growth. Do not rub or wash your nipples. Instead, gently pat off any milk with a dry cloth or, if a large amount of milk has leaked onto your breast, gently remove it with a cloth moistened with clear water. In addition, you can cleanse your breasts once a day in the shower, allowing the water to slowly stream over them. Avoid the use of soap on your nipples, since it will remove protective oils and dry the skin.

While some mothers believe that the use of breast creams will improve the health of the breast tissue, such lotions and ointments have never been shown to be beneficial, even when soreness develops. See Chapter 15 for a discussion of lubricants.

If you are using breast pads to absorb leaking milk, be certain to remove all plastic layers that can trap moisture next to your skin. If leaking milk has dried, causing your bra or breast pads to stick to your skin, first moisten the area for easy removal. Pulling the dry material off like a bandage may remove layers of skin and damage delicate tissues.

Taking all of these precautions will help to preserve the health of your breasts, making breastfeeding enjoyable for you and your baby. As you become more experienced, sound breastfeeding management practices will become second nature to you, and nursings will take less time. You will then be able to turn your full attention to your baby's changing needs and take even greater pleasure in his growth and development.

AT A GLANCE

Getting Off to the Best Possible Start

Preparing to Nurse

- Set up a routine for nursings.
- Prepare yourself, and gather appropriate items in your nursing spot.
- Rouse or calm your baby, as needed.
- Relax with your baby to ensure letdown.

Establishing a Pattern for Getting Your Baby on Your Breast

- Hold your baby close to you, tummy to tummy, with his mouth aligned slightly below the center of your breast.
- Mold your nipple between your thumb and fingers.
- Brush against your baby's lips to stimulate rooting reflex.
- As your baby opens his mouth, insert your nipple and areola.
- If incorrectly positioned, remove your breast and try again.

Practicing Good Nursing Technique

- Check to ensure that your baby's mouth is well back on the breast, with his lips flanged outward and his tongue cupped around the areola.
- Nurse on the first side until your baby spontaneously releases the breast.
- Nurse on second side only as long as baby is interested.
- During the early weeks, nurse at least 9 times per day.
- During the first week, try to space daytime feedings no more than three hours apart.
- Burp your baby after nursing on each breast.
- Start each feeding with the alternate breast.

Maintaining Healthy Nipples

- Air dry your nipples after nursings to prevent soreness.
- Avoid using breast creams.
- Avoid plastic bra and pad liners that can trap moisture.
- Avoid the use of soap on your nipples.

7 Overcoming Temporary Roadblocks

Beginning life with a new baby can be an exhilarating experience—a time when all things are fresh and new. It can also be a confusing period, when you question your ability to be a good mother. This contrast of good and bad feelings confronts mothers every day. Happily, the pleasant experiences far outnumber the unpleasant ones. By using common sense, taking advantage of available information, and obtaining advice from those close to you, you will learn how to deal with problems as they arise.

Most women nurse their babies with little or no trouble, and the few difficulties that do arise are easily overcome. When these roadblocks make getting started difficult, however, breastfeeding can be frustrating and upsetting. You can minimize such problems and shorten their duration by understanding what causes the difficulties and learning how to treat them. Although some situations may seem overwhelming at first, keep in mind that most breastfeeding problems are temporary. After the initial difficulties have been resolved, you will be able to look forward to many months of success and enjoyment.

WHEN YOUR BABY HAS TROUBLE GRASPING THE NIPPLE

During the early days of nursing, many infants are only moderately successful in grasping the breast. Breastfeeding is a learned skill that requires a period of transition for both mother and baby. You can help your baby learn to grasp the breast by stimulating his rooting reflex. You may also have to adjust your baby's position at the breast, moving him closer so that his mouth is aligned slightly below the center of the breast. By using the C-hold, you will be able to support your breast without experiencing discomfort or strain.

Occasionally, a condition exists that makes grasping the breast unusually difficult. Some situations arise from the baby's medical condition or from his confusion about the suckling process, while others result from the physical nature of the nipple.

Infant-Related Problems

The length of time that passes between birth and the first feeding can influence your baby's initial ability to grasp your nipple and begin to nurse. A baby's natural suckling instincts are strongest during the first six hours of life. For this reason, contact between mother and baby should ideally take place directly after birth. A premature birth or a birth in which medications are administered can diminish the baby's initial ability to suckle. An underdeveloped sucking reflex is another condition that can complicate early feedings. These are all problems that, although frustrating for both you and your baby, are temporary in nature and will be remedied by the passage of time.

Occasionally, a medical condition exists that requires special breastfeeding techniques. While a cleft lip may present a feeding challenge, your baby will be able to grasp the nipple if you cover the cleft with your finger or your breast while nursing. A mentally handicapped baby may have difficulty remembering how to suckle, and will therefore require constant reteaching. Such obstacles can be overcome with patience and a positive outlook. While breastfeeding may not follow the usual course, a successful and fulfilling experience can be enjoyed.

Incorrect Tongue Positioning

For nursing to be successful, the baby's tongue must be positioned between his lower gum and the underside of the breast. The breast is then compressed in a wave-like motion against the roof of the mouth, with pressure starting at the tip of the tongue and rolling backwards. The baby's gums work with his tongue to squeeze the milk out.

Some babies, although able to grasp the breast and maintain suction, incorrectly position the tongue when trying to nurse. When a baby pulls the back portion of his tongue up, he is unable to extract milk from the breast. Moreover, a baby may press his tongue against the roof of his mouth, blocking the opening and making nursing impossible. Sometimes, too, a baby may close his mouth just as the mother tries to insert her breast, and consequently grasp only the end of the nipple.

You can use a simple technique to check your baby's tongue position. During a feeding, gently pull down his lower lip. His tongue should cover the lower gum line and curve around the nipple. If it is difficult for you to evaluate his sucking during a feeding, you can use another method. When your baby is not nursing, brush his lips so that he opens his mouth, and gently place the pad of your finger against his soft palate. His tongue should curve around your finger and stroke backwards. If your baby's tongue blocks your finger, or if the sucking motion is in reverse, you may need to correct your baby's sucking technique. Other signs of a problem are gagging when the finger is only slightly inserted, frustration at the beginning of a feeding, and a need to nurse constantly. If your baby has difficulty sucking, try to hold his tongue down as you insert your breast.

Nipple Confusion

Another possible cause of a baby's difficulty in grasping the nipple is confusion between your nipple and a bottle nipple. In bottle feeding, suction causes milk to flow out of the nipple openings, and the tongue is used to stop the flow—a process that is basically the reverse of breastfeeding (see Figure 7.1). If a newborn baby is alternately offered bottle and breast, he is likely to become confused by the two different methods of obtaining milk.

In breastfeeding, the tongue thrusts upwards and forwards to grasp the breast. The gums squeeze the areola and the tongue compresses the breast backwards in a wave-like motion, creating negative pressure for suction. Lips are flanged outward around the breast. Cheek muscles assist.

In bottle feeding, the tongue thrusts upwards to control milk flow. Gums and lips cannot create compression. Air flows freely. Facial muscles are relaxed.

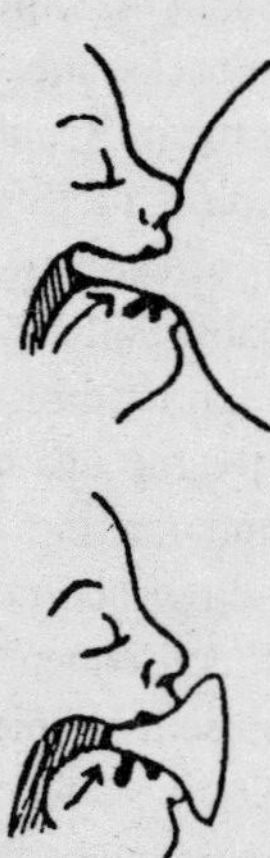

Figure 7.1 Methods of Sucking on Bottle and Breast

To avoid creating sucking confusion for your baby, delay introducing a bottle into your baby's feeding routine as long as possible. If there is a medical need for supplements, or if a return to work cannot be postponed, additional nourishment can be offered in a nursing supplementer, spoon, eyedropper, or small cup. If you must offer a bottle, delay it until breastfeeding has become firmly established—at about six to eight weeks.

Nipple-Related Problems

The nature of the nipple itself may cause your baby problems.

Perhaps the tissue surrounding it is inflexible and cannot be stretched easily, or the nipple is flat or inverted. (See page 20 for a description of these variations in nipples.) If your nipples do not protrude enough for your baby to grasp them easily, you can perform the Hoffman technique described on page 21. Before feedings, the nipple can be molded by hand or stimulated with ice to make it more erect. Sometimes, a manual or electric breast pump can be used to draw the nipple out just before the baby is put to the breast. Whenever you are not nursing, you can wear breast shells during the day to train your nipples to extend outward.

As a last resort, a special device can be worn at the beginning of feedings. This device, the nipple shield, is an artificial nipple that is placed over the mother's nipple. As the baby sucks on the artificial device, the mother's nipple is drawn out. When used correctly, the shield is removed immediately after the baby has drawn the nipple out, and the baby nurses directly on the mother's breast for the rest of the feeding. Because use of a nipple shield can introduce other problems, as explained on page 218, caution is advised.

WHEN YOU THINK YOUR BREASTS ARE ENGORGED

Frequently, postpartum breast fullness is mistaken for engorgement. However, postpartum fullness is a normal condition that accompanies the initial production of breast milk. Engorgement, on the other hand, is a condition of overfullness that results from an inadequate emptying of the breast. It is important to understand the distinction between these two conditions so that proper action can be taken in each instance.

The Characteristics of Normal Fullness

Shortly after delivery, the amount of blood circulating in your breasts will begin to increase. This will serve as the source of your first milk. As the blood is utilized and broken down, additional lymph (a clear, alkaline fluid in the lymphatic vessels) is produced to carry away the unused components of the blood. As your breasts begin making true milk on the second or third day after delivery, they will start to feel tight and full from the increased amounts of blood and lymph. You may even see the enlarged blood vessels under the surface of your skin. If your bra seems to be pressing on the tissues, a larger bra or the use of a bra extender may help to relieve your discomfort.

The normal lactating breast is soft and pliable, even when full of milk. However, in the early days of nursing, fullness and a small degree of tenderness is common. With frequent nursings, the fullness will gradually subside, finally disappearing about ten days after delivery. As this fullness diminishes, some women worry that they may be losing their milk supply. The loss of fullness, however, reflects a decrease in the extra fluids and enlarged blood supply that accompanied the initial production of milk.

Detecting True Engorgement

Engorgement is a condition of overfullness that occurs when the breasts are not emptied well enough or often enough. It can begin soon after birth if colostrum is not cleared from the duct system, or any time the breasts are not emptied sufficiently. You will know that your breasts are engorged when you experience considerable pain, and your breasts feel hard, warm, and tender to the touch. The skin may appear taut, shiny, and transparent, and your nipples may become tender and seem flat in contrast to the swelling of the surrounding tissues.

When engorgement develops, the flow of blood and lymph is inhibited by the increased pressure of milk in the ducts. The pressure also makes fewer nutrients available for the production of milk and decreases the ability of the alveoli to produce milk. As blood and lymph build up, breast tissues swell, preventing bacteria and cell particles from being removed properly and increasing the chance of infection. In addition, the enlargement of the breast tissues may make your nipples difficult to grasp, causing your baby to nurse on the end of the nipples. Such incorrect suckling results in sore or cracked nipples and fails to stimulate the nipples enough to ensure letdown and maintain milk production.

Preventing Engorgement

In light of the many complications that can arise from engorgement, care should be taken to prevent its occurrence. You can avoid engorgement by removing milk from your breasts whenever they feel full or when feedings are missed, either through nursing or through hand expression or pumping. Regular, frequent feedings will prevent your breasts from becoming overly full between feedings. Be sure to nurse long enough each time to remove most of the milk from the first breast, and to alternate the breast with which you start each feeding.

Relieving Engorgement

If your breasts become engorged, you may need to nurse more frequently for a while (every one and a half to two hours) until the fullness and pain disappear. Prior to feedings, you can hand express or pump milk for a short time to draw out the nipple, thus making it easier to grasp. Apply warm compresses to your breasts before feedings to increase blood circulation and milk flow; then apply cold compresses after feedings to reduce circulation and relieve pain. If nursing does not empty your breasts, stand in a warm shower or bathe your breasts in warm water, gently massaging and hand expressing to relieve fullness. Because breast tissues swell during engorgement, the pain may subside more slowly than the fullness.

WHEN YOUR NIPPLES BECOME SORE

At times, the enjoyment and rewards of nursing are delayed because of discomfort from initial nipple soreness. Although correct prenatal care of your nipples, proper positioning of your baby at the breast, and the avoidance of irritants can help to minimize nipple soreness, such measures may not totally prevent it. Your nipples need to become accustomed to the pulling and stress of nursing, and you will probably experience some tenderness until layers of tough, protective skin develop. If soreness does occur, a number of effective treatments are available.

Preventing Prolonged Nipple Soreness

Nipple soreness can be caused by poor nursing habits, improper breast care, or a number of physical conditions. However, the major cause of nipple soreness is incorrect positioning of the baby's mouth on the breast. When the breast is far back in the baby's mouth, the nipple is pulled back to the soft palate where it is not subject to strong pressure from the tongue. The collecting sinuses beneath the areola are compressed with a wave-like motion, moving the milk out of the nipple. When the breast is farther forward in the baby's mouth, the sinuses are not compressed to the same degree, and milk does not come out as readily. In addition, the tongue compresses the nipple against the hard palate, causing abrasion. Your own comfort level should help you assess your baby's nursing position. When your baby nurses, you should not feel pain.

Another indicator of poor positioning is the appearance of the baby's mouth and cheeks. In a good nursing position, your baby's mouth will be open wide, with his lips flanged outward, his nose and chin touching your breast, and his cheeks appearing normally rounded and full. In a poor nursing position, your baby's lips will be pursed and not so widely opened; his cheeks will appear hollow and will move inward and outward in an effort to compensate for the lesser amount of breast tissue in his mouth.

Once nipple soreness begins to develop, it can be halted by improving the position of the baby's mouth on the breast. Using another body position may also promote more rapid healing, as the placement of the baby's tongue and palate will be on a different area of the breast. Alternating between the cradle, football, and lying-down nursing positions will decrease stress on any one area of the breast.

By following the suggestions listed in Table 7.1 and using

common sense, you will either avoid nipple soreness or greatly reduce the duration of the problem.

Remedies for Sore Nipples

Sore nipples that remain untreated can develop cracks or blisters that require a lengthy healing time. When used at the first sign of soreness, the remedies listed in Table 7.2 will bring noticeable relief within twenty-four to forty-eight hours, helping you avoid more severe discomfort. If your nipples have been sore for several days, healing may take a bit longer. The important thing to keep in mind is that nipple soreness is temporary! Prompt action will help to relieve the discomfort so that you can enjoy breastfeeding without pain.

A Word About Thrush

A few women experience persistently sore nipples that fail to respond to the usual treatment. Often, such soreness is the result of thrush, a yeast infection to which many babies are exposed during the birth process. When thrush organisms are present in the newborn's system, they may later be transmitted from the baby's mouth to the mother's nipples. Thrush can appear as white patches on your nipples and in your baby's mouth, or as red pimples or a red rash on your baby's skin in the diaper area. However, these symptoms are not always obvious. If you experience persistently sore nipples, you and your baby may both have thrush. Without proper treatment, thrush can continue indefinitely; with proper medical treatment, it responds quickly.

If you suspect that thrush is present, contact either your own doctor or your baby's doctor. You will probably be given a prescription for the antibiotic nystatin, which comes in two forms. Mycostatin is swabbed on the nipples and mouth, while Mycolog is applied to the skin in the diaper area. In order to totally eliminate the infection, be sure to use the medications for the entire period prescribed by your doctor. You and your baby must be treated simultaneously so that you do not pass the infec-

Table 7.1 Causes and Prevention of Sore Nipples

Causes	Prevention
• Normal postpartum fullness.	• Feed frequently.
• Nipple is stretched during nursing.	• Hold baby closely, positioned on his side facing you.
• Breast is not positioned well in baby's mouth.	• Align baby's mouth slightly below nipple center, well back onto breast, with baby's nose and chin touching breast and his lips flanged outward.
• Baby is held in the same position at every feeding.	• Vary nursing positions often to avoid stress on any one area of the breast.
• Baby chews onto or off of the nipple at feedings.	• Use care in putting baby on and off nipple correctly.
• Baby nurses vigorously from overhunger, low milk supply, or poor letdown.	• Nurse frequently, use relaxation techniques, and hand express milk to initiate letdown.
• A nipple shield is worn for the entire feeding.	• Use shield only to start feeding, then remove it.
• Natural lubrication has been removed from nipple.	• Avoid use of soap and drying agents on breasts.
• Nipple skin is damaged, irritated, or lacks resilience due to improper clothing or plastic in pads.	• Use proper nipple care, avoid fabrics that hold moisture, and vary nursing positions.
• Breast shells are worn continuously between feedings.	• Wear shells only for short periods.
• Unbalanced diet has led to poor skin condition.	• Select foods from the four food groups at every meal.
• You are menstruating or pregnant.	• Nipple soreness is only temporary.

tion back and forth. To prevent a recurrence of the problem, it is a good idea to discard any bottle nipples, pacifiers, and teething rings your baby has used.

Table 7.2 Remedies for Sore Nipples

Time	Treatment
Before Feedings	• Use relaxation techniques. • Massage your breasts. • Express some milk to encourage let-down and eliminate vigorous sucking. • Rub ice on the end of your nipple to numb it directly before inserting it into your baby's mouth. This may sound uncomfortable, but it isn't! • If a blister has formed, soak your nipple with a warm moist compress to soften it before nursing.
During Feedings	• Use correct nursing position. • Nurse your baby more frequently. • Limit nursing time on the sore nipple. • Nurse on the least sore side first to avoid vigorous suckling at the beginning of the feeding. • Position your baby so that his chin is opposite the sore area.
After Feedings	• Air dry your nipples thoroughly. • Apply a breast cream after air drying. See page 217 for a discussion of lubricants and their correct use.
Between Feedings	• To aid healing, soak your nipples in a solution of 1/4 teaspoon salt and 8 ounces of water for 10 to 15 minutes.

WHEN JAUNDICE DEVELOPS

About 50 percent of full-term infants and 75 percent of premature infants develop jaundice. **Jaundice**, which is often a sign that the baby's system is immature, is characterized by a yellow coloring to the skin. In more severe cases, the baby may suffer from weakness or a loss of appetite. Jaundice occurs when fetal red blood cells break down normally, but the body cannot excrete them quickly enough and they accumulate as a substance called **bilirubin**. A large number of drugs when given to the mother late in pregnancy or during lactation have been linked to increased jaundice in the baby. Some substances, such as caffeine and oxytocin, are a subject of controversy. Others have been proven to contribute to jaundice. These include the salicylates, the sulfonamides, Vitamin K, the thiazides, novobiocin, and diazepam.[1]

It has been found that babies who nurse frequently from birth (at least nine times a day) have a lower incidence of jaundice than those who are fed less frequently.[2] Early, frequent nursings will help your baby to excrete meconium, the thick substance that constitutes a baby's first bowel movements. The passage of meconium, which has a high concentration of bilirubin, will reduce your baby's bilirubin level. Frequent nursings will also provide your baby with more fluids, increase the number of bowel movements, and reduce the recirculation of bilirubin.

There are several types of jaundice, including physiologic jaundice, pathologic jaundice, and breast milk jaundice. The characteristics and recommended treatments of each form are discussed on the following pages.

Physiologic Jaundice

To identify which of the various forms of jaundice is present, doctors observe the infant's bilirubin level. In common newbaby jaundice—*physiologic jaundice*—the bilirubin level usually rises slowly, reaches a peak by the third day, remains elevated for several days, and falls by the end of the first week. With this type of jaundice, the bilirubin levels remain within a safe range, far below the danger level associated with serious problems like weakness and loss of appetite.

Medical opinions vary concerning acceptable bilirubin levels, as well as methods for treating jaundice. Generally, however, a bilirubin level between 1 and 8 milligrams (mg) is considered safe for a normal newborn infant. Most physicians will begin treatment if the level rises above the range of 10 to 12 mg. A level of 20 mg is considered dangerous for full-term newborns. Jaundice is more common in premature babies because of the body's immaturity. Since a premie is unable to process bilirubin well, his acceptable bilirubin levels are much lower.

The Treatment of Physiologic Jaundice

In order for your baby's bilirubin level to decline, the by-products of redblood-cell breakdown must be eliminated from his body. Because sunlight helps to break down bilirubin, your doctor may advise you to expose as much of your baby's skin as possible to sunlight. In most hospital settings, sunlight can be simulated through the use of special fluorescent **"bili" lights**. For maximum exposure, the baby is fully unclothed, and his eyes are shielded to protect them from the rays.

If your baby receives treatment under "bili" lights, you can ask that the lights be brought to your room so that you can continue nursings, or you can request to visit the nursery for feedings. As a result of your baby's exposure to the "bili" lights, he may be sluggish and temporarily unable to suck well. Other possible side effects of the "bili" lights are dehydration, loose stools, and a skin rash. These symptoms will disappear after the treatment is stopped. Short, frequent feedings will help your baby to nurse while he is undergoing treatment. Many times, babies are given extra fluids in an attempt to flush the excess bilirubin from their systems. Supplementary fluids, however, have been shown to be of no help in lowering bilirubin levels. [3]

Pathologic Jaundice, A Cause for Concern

When bilirubin levels are found to be quite high, either at the time of birth or shortly thereafter, **pathologic jaundice** is usually suspected. This type of jaundice is due to disease, the dysfunction of an organ, or a condition such as Rh incompatibility. Sometimes, what was thought to be physiologic jaundice is discovered to be pathologic jaundice when low bilirubin levels suddenly rise above a critical level.

The Treatment of Pathologic Jaundice

Pathologic jaundice can cause brain damage and even death if it is not treated appropriately. "Bili" lights and blood transfusions may be used to lower bilirubin levels. Depending on the severity of the condition, breastfeeding may be suspended until the baby is out of danger. Pathologic jaundice is fairly uncommon, however, affecting only a small percentage of infants. When it does occur, the success rate for treatment is extremely high.

Breast Milk Jaundice

Some doctors order mothers to stop nursing when jaundice occurs. This practice stems from a concern that the baby is suffering from **breast milk jaundice**, a condition believed to be caused by a component of the mothers breast milk. Breast milk jaundice, however, is extremely rare, occurring in less than one percent of all cases.

Breast milk jaundice differs from physiologic jaundice in that it develops more slowly, not beginning until *four to seven days after birth.* It then peaks between ten to fourteen days, and may last as long as six weeks. It is unlikely, therefore, that jaundice diagnosed in the first three days after birth has been caused by the mother's breast milk.

The Treatment of Breast Milk Jaundice

Even when the presence of breast milk jaundice is suspected, some experts feel that it is unnecessary to suspend breastfeeding. Instead, they prefer to try the methods used to treat physiologic jaundice. If your doctor instructs you to stop nursing, request a short delay to see if the bilirubin level can be reduced by other means.

If a suspension of nursing is prescribed, however, it need not be permanent. You will probably be asked to refrain from nursing for one to four days to speed the removal of bilirubin. During that time, you will be able to maintain your milk supply by expressing milk regularly. You can also ask for frequent checks of your baby's bilirubin level so that nursing can be resumed as soon as possible.

Questions to Ask Your Doctor About Jaundice

Jaundice—like any infant illness—may make you feel confused and anxious. Reduce emotional stress by spending as much time as possible with your baby. Just seeing and holding him may make you feel better. Ask that treatment take place in your hospital room, and that you and your baby be allowed periods of eye and skin contact. Most important, keep in mind that infant jaundice is extremely common, and that it can be treated with great success. To become better informed about your baby's condition and treatment, ask your doctor the following questions:

- What tests have been done and what are the results?
- How long will the jaundice last?
- How often can the baby be nursed?
- If breastfeeding has been stopped, when can it be resumed?
- When will the baby be able to go home?

By keeping informed of your baby's progress and working with your doctor to develop a care plan that allows frequent feedings, you will be able to maintain your milk supply while providing the best possible care for your child. Although jaundice may initially be frightening, the period of treatment will pass quickly, and you and your family will soon be able to enjoy the love and security of being together.

WHEN NURSING IS SUSPENDED

At some time, you may be unable to nurse your baby for a day or more, perhaps because of hospitalization, the use of a medication, or a social weekend. With proper management, you will be able to meet your baby's nutritional needs, ensure your own well-being, and reestablish breastfeeding when desired.

Prepare for the event as far in advance as possible so that you will have time to become accustomed to pumping and expressing your milk. (See Chapter 15 for instructions on expressing and collecting milk.) Every day, try to collect enough extra milk for one feeding. You can freeze this expressed milk so that it can be given to your baby while you are gone. To ensure that your baby will accept feedings from a bottle, the person who will be caring for your baby should offer him an occasional bottle before the separation.

To maintain your milk supply and avoid the discomfort of overfullness during the separation, be sure to pump or express your milk regularly, possibly following the schedule you use for nursings. Be alert to any symptoms of engorgement or plugged ducts, and deal with them at the first sign of a problem. See this chapter for ways of treating engorgement, and Chapter 8 for suggestions on handling plugged ducts.

When you resume nursing, you may find that your milk supply has decreased. Rebuild it by increasing nursings and reducing the number of supplementary feedings. Depending on his age, your baby may be reluctant to nurse, or may seem distant. Give him lots of loving attention as you gradually return to your former nursing pattern.

AT A GLANCE

Overcoming Temporary Roadblocks

Baby's Ability to Grasp the Nipple

- Difficulty in grasping the nipple can be caused by flat or inverted nipples, engorgement, prematurity, medications, a delayed first nursing, incorrect sucking, or nipple confusion.
- To make your nipple more graspable, use the Hoffman technique, mold the nipple by hand, stimulate the nipple with ice, or draw out the nipple with a breast pump, breast shells, or — as a last resort — a nipple shield.

Engorgement

- Engorgement is characterized by hard, tender breasts that appear shiny and transparent.
- To avoid engorgement, empty your breasts regularly, pumping when the baby fails to empty the breast at feedings.
- Treat engorgement with warm compresses before nursings, cold compresses after nursings, and more frequent feedings.

Preventing Prolonged Nipple Soreness

- Breastfeeding should not hurt!
- To avoid stressing any one area of the nipple, vary nursing positions often.
- Position your baby correctly, supporting him as needed.
- Put your baby on and off the breast correctly.
- To avoid vigorous nursings caused by overhunger or a low milk supply, nurse frequently.
- Avoid the use of cleansing agents that can remove the nipple's natural lubricants.
- Avoid the incorrect use of a nipple shield.
- To improve your resistance to disease, follow a sound diet.
- Learn to identify thrush, initiating appropriate treatment when necessary.

Relieving Nipple Soreness

- Check position of baby at breast.
- Nurse more frequently.
- Nurse on the least sore side first.
- Limit nursing time on the sore nipple.
- Position your baby so his chin is opposite the sore area.
- Vary nursing positions often.
- Massage your breasts and express milk to encourage letdown.
- Rub ice on the end of the nipple before nursing.
- Air dry your nipples after every feeding. Soak the sore nipple in a solution of salt and water.

Jaundice

- Jaundice occurs when fetal red blood cells accumulate in the baby's body.
- There are three forms of jaundice: physiologic, pathologic, and breast milk.
- Frequent nursings beginning at birth can help reduce the likelihood of jaundice.
- For the safety of the baby, jaundice should be treated promptly.
- Breast milk jaundice is rare. Usually, breast milk is *not* the cause of infant jaundice.
- In the event of jaundice, weaning is usually unnecessary.
- If suspended breastfeeding is prescribed, it need not be permanent.

Suspended Breastfeeding

- Prepare for the event in advance by expressing and saving milk.
- Have the person who will care for your baby offer him an occasional bottle ahead of time.
- Until nursing resumes, express your milk to relieve fullness.
- When nursing resumes, rebuild your milk supply through frequent feedings.

8

Making Physical Adjustments to Childbirth and Breastfeeding

The lifestyle of many American women today does not prepare them for the rigors of childbirth. Pregnancy and childbirth make demands on the body that require a time of recovery and adjustment.

Breastfeeding, too, requires a period of adjustment. As your body changes to meet the nutritional needs of your infant, you will have to adapt to the changes within your body. Most of what you experience will be normal and natural. Leaking, for instance, is quite common, and need not be a source of concern. Some conditions, however, are not only troublesome, but can be avoided. Plugged ducts and breast infections, for instance, are the result of improper breastfeeding management. Be assured that these problems—as well as those resulting from childbirth—can be treated successfully, and that you will, in time, regain a feeling of well-being.

YOUR RECOVERY FROM CHILDBIRTH

Don't be surprised if you are a little tired and uncomfortable after giving birth. Delivering a baby is a most extraordinary and strenuous task. Whether you deliver vaginally or by Cesarean, you should expect some aftereffects. A period of recovery will be needed in order for your body to return to its prepregnant size and shape. Understandably, you will want to get back into your favorite clothes as soon as possible. Keep in mind, though, that the body undergoes nine months of changes during pregnancy. Allow yourself at least the same amount of time to return to your prepregnant condition.

Physical Changes After Delivery

Realistically, there will be many physical adjustments during the weeks following your baby's birth. Few women fit the blissful image of a new mother as she is portrayed in media advertising. The abdominal muscles and pelvic ligaments must stretch during pregnancy to accommodate the growing fetus; after your baby is born, it will take time and exercise for them to regain their firmness. After birth, your abdomen will still protrude slightly, and you may temporarily retain a waddle in your walk because of loose pelvic ligaments. Walking may also be hindered by the large sanitary pads that are worn to absorb the lochia discharge. If you have had an episiotomy, walking and sitting may cause you discomfort. Your breasts, also, may be uncomfortable due to the fullness caused by initial milk production. Perhaps this is not what you expected, but at least you will know that you are not alone!

Soon after birth, your body will begin the healing process. Within about six weeks, your uterus will shrink from its predelivery weight of two pounds to its prepregnant weight of about two ounces. You may experience some afterpains from the contractions that accompany this decrease in the size of your uterus. The nipple stimulation experienced during breastfeeding will help to quicken the process by contracting the uterus even more, thus reducing the possibility of excessive bleeding. Because of this relationship between breastfeeding and uterine contractions, your afterpains may grow more intense when your baby is suckling at your breast.

Pamper Yourself!

Be kind to yourself after delivery, allowing your body to recuperate from the experience of giving birth. You cannot expect to resume your previous activity level immediately after having a baby (regardless of what is said about pioneer women giving birth and returning to work in the fields hours later!). Rest is essential for milk production, the rebuilding of tissues, and—perhaps most important—a sense of wellbeing. When you feel good, your outlook will be more positive and you will be better able to cope with new situations. Lack of proper rest can result in excessive bleeding, exhaustion, dizziness, a weak pelvic floor, sore nipples, and breast infections. This is not meant to scare you, but to convince you of your need to limit activities during the first few weeks after delivery.

This advice to rest may not always be practical, especially with all the demands of family, household, and work. If you are raising your child alone, these demands will be even greater. But try to get as much rest as possible. If you stay at home in your bathrobe for a couple of weeks after delivery, you not only will discourage visitors from staying too long, but probably will be less inclined to pursue as many activities as you would if you were fully dressed. To get additional rest, lie down during nursings. After your baby has been well-fed and settled in his bed, take advantage of the lull by napping yourself.

Until you feel more rested and able to resume household tasks, you may need to put up with a little more clutter and mess around the house. Don't worry about visitors seeing a messy house. They are there to see you and your baby, not your home. You may even find that friends and relatives are willing to help with some of your tasks, such as shopping for groceries, running errands, fixing dinner, and doing laundry—the possibilities are endless! If you have no one to help you and are really bothered by the clutter, do only those chores that annoy you most, and learn to leave others undone for a few weeks.

Your baby's demands on your time will decrease as he gets

older, so the feeling that your time is totally occupied by your baby is only temporary. Indulge yourself by totally enjoying your baby while you have the excuse and the opportunity. There will plenty of time to resume responsibilities later.

CHANGES IN YOUR BREASTS

During the months that you are breastfeeding, you may become aware of a number of different changes in your breasts. Your breasts will feel very different from the way they did before pregnancy. Most evident will be the normal lumpy nature of the lactating breast, which you will notice when you perform your monthly breast self-examinations. If you are not already performing regular breast exams, now is the time to begin. It is best to do these exams just after a feeding, when your breasts are empty. If you have begun menstruating, it is preferable to wait until your period ends, since it will temporarily alter breast fullness and texture. Figure 8.1 explains the correct procedure for performing a breast self-exam.

Fibrocystic Disease

During breast examinations, you may notice lumps that do not seem to be a part of the normal lumpiness associated with breastfeeding. This may be a sign of **fibrocystic disease**, a condition in which nonmalignant lumps appear within the breast tissue. Fibrocystic disease is extremely common in varying degrees among women. Aching and tenderness is associated with the condition, which frequently becomes more noticeable prior to menstruation, and may also be pronounced while your are breastfeeding.

By becoming familiar with the normal nature of your breasts, especially during breastfeeding, you will learn to detect changes in texture. You can reduce the severity of fibrocystic disease by eliminating caffeine from your diet[1] and, according to some doctors, by taking daily supplements of Vitamin E.[2]

While fibrocystic disease is common—and, in and of itself, is not dangerous—you should always consult your doctor when

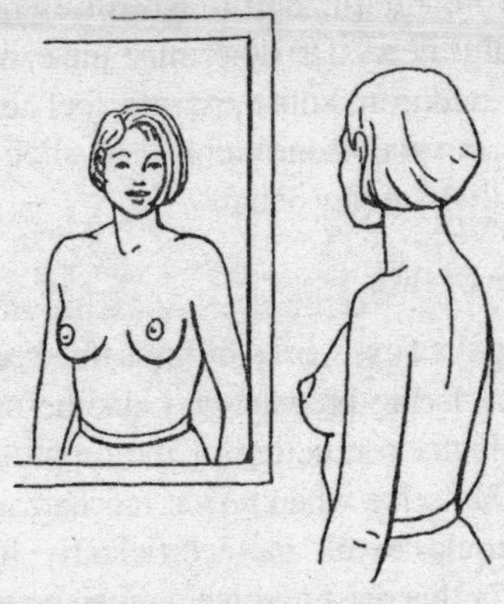

Examine your breasts regularly to check for any lump, hard knot, or thickening. Learn to recognize the normal contours of your breasts, and ask your doctor to confirm your findings during your next visit. If you feel any new lumps or any lumps that have enlarged, promptly report this to your doctor.

1. Look at your breasts in the mirror, first with your arms at your sides, and then with your arms above your head. Look for changes in the appearance of the breasts or nipples, such as a swelling or dimpling of the skin.

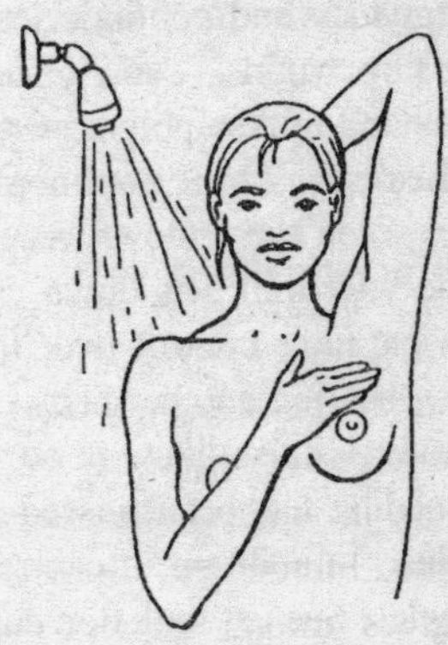

2. Place your arms at your side. Keeping your fingers flat, gently palpate one breast with the opposite hand by moving the hand in a circular motion over the entire breast area. You may wish to do this during a bath or shower, as your fingers will then glide easily over the wet skin. Repeat the procedure on the second breast. Then, with arms raised, repeat the procedure again. While your arms are raised, carefully palpate the nipple area and the tissue lying under it.

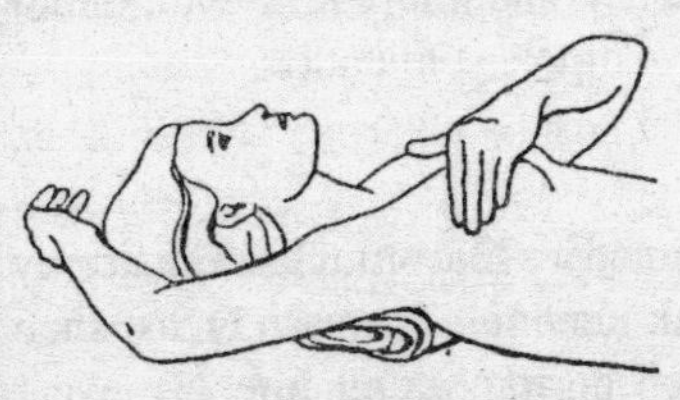

3. Lie flat on your back with a pillow or folded towel placed under your shoulder on the first side that is to be examined. Using the same circular motion described earlier, check the texture of your breast. Move the towel or pillow to the other shoulder, and repeat the procedure.

Figure 8.1 Breast Self-Examination

you discover any lumps in your breast. Self-diagnosis is not always accurate; a professional is needed to determine the exact nature of any irregularity. In addition, some experts feel that fibrocystic disease may lead to other conditions, and should therefore be monitored carefully by a physician.

When Milk Leaks From Your Breasts

Many women leak milk during the first weeks of breastfeeding, and some even leak colostrum during pregnancy. Leaking is a normal part of lactation. The interior structure of the nipple is composed mostly of muscles that serve as a closing mechanism for the milk ducts. These muscles work more efficiently for some women than for others. For this reason, some women never experience leaking, while others begin leaking colostrum during pregnancy and continue leaking milk for months after breastfeeding begins. Usually, however, leaking subsides after the mother's milk supply adjusts itself to her baby's needs.

Leaking is quite common during the early days of breastfeeding, when the letdown reflex is being established. In fact, any time your milk lets down, leaking may occur, and you will not always have control over the letdown. Cuddling your baby or even hearing another baby cry may trigger your letdown reflex. Leaking is also likely to occur directly before a nursing or when a feeding has been missed—times when your breasts are their fullest. In addition, it can result from an overstimulation of the nipples. Such stimulation can accompany snack nursings—short feedings given to comfort or quiet the baby between regular, complete nursings. Sexual activity and the overuse of breast shells can also produce excessive nipple stimulation.

How to Avoid Leaking

To avoid leaking, discontinue practices that stimulate the nerves in your nipples. Eliminate snack nursings, decrease breast shell use, and limit breast stimulation during sexual foreplay. Wear loose clothing to prevent any unnecessary pressure on your breasts. If you are on medication, check with your physician to make sure that he has not prescribed any drugs that have the side effect of stimulating milk production. If any feedings are missed, remove milk from your breasts by manual expression or pumping to avoid overfullness. If leaking becomes a problem for you and your mate when you are making love, try nursing your baby before you have sexual relations.

When leaking does occur, there are a number of measures you can take to control or conceal it. Place temporary pressure on your breasts by pressing them with the palms of your hands or crossing your arms against your chest until the leaking stops. (See Figure 8.2.) Wearing a pad to absorb leaking milk will prevent your clothing from getting wet, while a towel can be used to protect bedding at night. Loosefitting, patterned clothing will conceal moisture, as will a sweater that is worn over your bodice.

While your baby is nursing on one breast, a plastic breast shell can be used to collect leaking milk from the other breast. This milk can be saved, provided that the shell has been sterilized prior to the feeding and the milk is refrigerated immediately at the end of the feeding. Many women find that leaking stops within the first six weeks after delivery. For a small number of women, however, leaking continues for many months. These women learn to anticipate when leaking is most likely to occur and to use the techniques described above to control it.

How to Manage Leaking

When leaking does occur, there are a number of measures you can take to control or conceal it. Place temporary pressure on your breasts by pressing them with the palms of your hands or crossing your arms against your chest until the leaking stops. (See Figure 8.2.) Wearing a pad to absorb leaking milk will prevent your clothing from getting wet, while a towel can be used to protect bedding at night. Loose-fitting, patterned clothing will conceal moisture, as will a sweater that is worn over your bodice.

While your baby is nursing on one breast, a plastic breast shell can be used to collect leaking milk from the other breast.

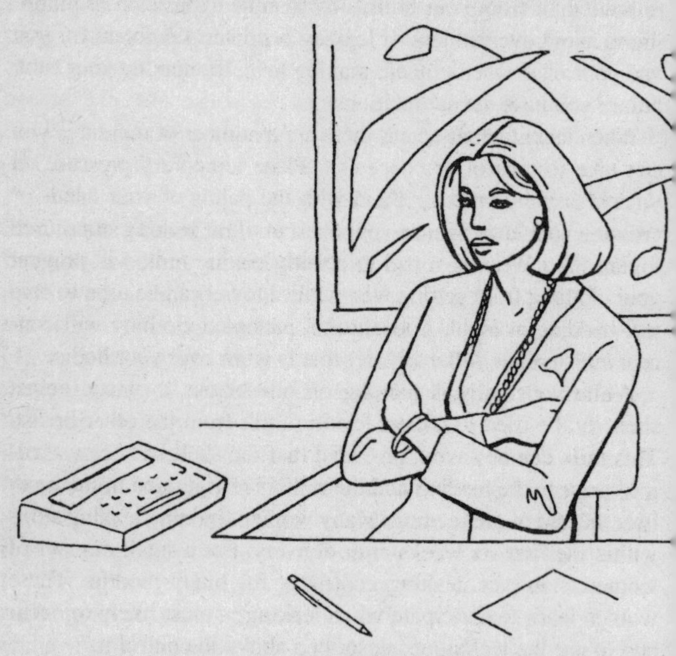

Figure 8.2 Controlling Leaking

This milk can be saved, provided that the shell has been sterilized prior to the feeding and the milk is refrigerated immediately at the end of the feeding. Many women find that leaking stops within the first six weeks after delivery. For a small number of women, however, leaking continues for many months. These women learn to anticipate when leaking is most likely to occur and to use the techniques described above to control it.

POSSIBLE BREAST PROBLEMS

While lumpiness and leaking are essentially normal occurrences, some types of breast changes are caused by the improper management of breastfeeding. Plugged ducts and breast infections are both direct results of an insufficient emptying of the milk ducts. They can be caused by missed feedings, poor positioning of the baby at the breast, inadequate nursing times at each breast, or pressure placed on portions of the breast. Breast infections may have external causes as well.

Plugged Ducts

When a milk duct becomes blocked by a thickened mass of milk or castoff cells, the resulting condition is termed a **plugged duct**. Characterized by local tenderness, lumpiness, or swelling, plugged ducts are caused by an incomplete emptying of the breasts, missed feedings, or an irregular nursing pattern. By consistently using the same nursing position, you may prevent certain collecting sinuses from being completely emptied. Constant pressure on your breasts may also create a plug. Such pressure can be caused by a tight bra, a sweater or heavy gown that is bunched up under your arm while nursing, a habit of frequently holding your baby in the same position against your chest, or the practice of sleeping on your side or stomach.

If a plugged duct is not treated quickly, it can develop into a breast infection. Therefore, prompt diagnosis and treatment are essential. Once you locate a possible plugged duct, have your baby nurse on the affected breast frequently, offering it first at every feeding so that it will receive the strongest suckling. To work the plug down the duct so that it can be released, position your baby so that his chin is pointing toward the plug. This will allow the affected milk duct to be stroked by the baby's tongue during the nursing. Breast massage and the application of warm, moist compresses during and between feedings will also encourage drainage.

When a plug is released, it may appear as a thick, stringy, brownish or greenish mass. Usually, the baby spits out this thickened milk and then returns to nursing. Sometimes, however, the baby doesn't react to the plug, and the mother never sees it. For this reason, you may not be aware that the plug has disappeared until the tenderness in your breast begins to subside. If, after several days, the pain continues and you are unable to work the lump down, contact your doctor for medical treatment.

Breast Infections

A **breast infection**, referred to medically as **mastitis**, is an infection that occurs within the breast tissue. Usually, it does not come in contact with the milk. If an area of your breast becomes infected, it will be red, hot, and tender to the touch. You may feel as if you have the flu, with chills, fever, aches, and fatigue. It is common to feel tired and achy before the symptoms appear in your breast, so be watchful for these signs.

Breast infections are most prevalent during the first weeks of breastfeeding, when you begin overexerting yourself and become overly tired. Fatigue makes you more susceptible to bacteria that is passed to you by your baby or by other family members, as well as to bacteria that enters through a cracked nipple. An irregular nursing pattern, too, may open you to infection by causing milk to remain in your breasts and stressing the ducts. Another possible source of infection is a plugged duct that has gone untreated, resulting in the slowing or stoppage of milk flow and allowing bacteria to multiply in the stagnant milk.

Sometimes women get breast infections over and over again because they continue to be exposed to bacteria carried by other family members. If you experience recurrent infections despite correct nursing management, consult your doctor. Ask that a culture be taken of your milk, your baby's mouth, and other members of your family. This will enable the doctor to determine if the infection has an external cause, and to treat all the affected persons simultaneously.

If a breast infection remains untreated, it can develop into an **abscess**, which is a localized collection of pus caused by a lack of drainage. The result is a red, swollen, tender area on the breast, accompanied by such symptoms as fever, extreme fatigue, dizziness, nausea, and aching muscles. Contact your doctor immediately if you suspect a breast abscess. An abscessed breast requires immediate medical treatment with a prescribed antibiotic, and drainage of the abscess by surgical means. If you are asked to temporarily discontinue nursing from the affected breast, pump to relieve discomfort.

Treating a Breast Infection

It is clear that breast infections must be treated immediately in order to prevent further complications. Often, the flu-like symptoms that accompany a breast infection lead a woman to misinterpret her illness as a case of flu. If you develop any flu-like symptoms during the time you are breastfeeding, determine if there is any tenderness in your breasts. Keep checking your breasts periodically during the first twenty-four hours to ensure that no infection is present.

In treating a breast infection, it is important that your breasts be emptied regularly, and the most efficient way to empty them is to nurse your baby frequently. Apply warm, moist compresses to your breast before and during nursings and get *complete bed rest* until the symptoms disappear. The need for bed rest cannot be stressed enough. While it may be difficult for you to remain in bed for the entire time, try to cancel work and social commitments and to rest as much as possible for several days. Bed rest will greatly speed your recovery.

Report your infection to your doctor; you may be advised to take an antibiotic. There are many antibiotics that can be taken while you continue to breastfeed. You may also ask to receive a low dosage of medication over a long period of time to minimize the concentration of the drug in your milk. Be aware, however, that the drug may not be as effective in this form. Be sure to take all of the prescribed medication, even after your symptoms have disappeared, so that the infection will not recur in a few days.

Nursing During a Breast Infection

Sometimes, mothers are instructed to stop breastfeeding until a breast infection has been cleared up. Often, they are advised to refrain from nursing for the duration of their treatment under antibiotics. However, regular, complete emptying of the breasts is essential to the treatment of a breast infection. The suspension of breastfeeding could compound your problem and prolong the infection.

Most nonhospital breast infections come from bacteria in the baby's mouth or the home environment. Your baby will have already been exposed to these bacteria and will be receiving antibodies through your milk. Additionally, because the infection is not usually in the milk ducts themselves, it is not in the milk. Consequently, it is unlikely that nursing will pose any danger to your baby.

If you have been instructed to stop nursing because of a breast infection, ask your doctor why it is considered necessary. A 1975 study concluded that "lactation can and perhaps should be continued during treatment, as it may speed recovery and will not adversely affect the infant. Weaning in these circumstances may be emotionally traumatic to mother and baby. It can be delayed safely until both are naturally ready for this change."[3] A more recent study, conducted in 1984, reported that regular emptying of the breasts shortens the duration of symptoms and significantly improves the mother's response to treatment.[4]

WHEN MENSTRUATION RESUMES

Menstruation will resume anywhere from six weeks to eighteen months after your baby is born. Be advised that you could become fertile *before* you begin menstruating, so take precautions against an unwanted pregnancy. The timing of your first menstrual period will depend in part on the frequency of your nursings and the length of time you nurse your baby without supplemental feedings. Your baby's suckling will cause a high level of the hormone prolactin in your body. When a high level of prolactin is maintained through frequent nipple stimulation, ovulation is inhibited.

Many women begin menstruating soon after they have begun supplementing their baby's diet with formula or solid foods, since the baby then spends less time suckling at the breast. If you begin supplements and then discontinue them, you may even find that your menstrual periods will start up for a while and then stop again. Your baby's sleeping pattern, too, can affect menstruation. For instance, your first period may begin shortly after your baby begins sleeping for longer periods at night—and, in turn, eliminates night feedings. In fact, any change in your baby's nursing pattern, whether it increases or decreases the frequency of feedings, can affect your menstrual cycle.

After menstruation resumes, you can continue to nurse without harming your baby. Menstruation will not change the nutritional value of your milk. However, hormones can affect the taste of your milk, and your baby may be fussy or refuse to nurse on the days when you are menstruating. Such fussiness can also be a response to any emotional tension that you experience during menstruation. If your baby seems to reject breastfeeding during your menstrual period, try to be patient and understanding. Your nursing routine should return to normal at the end of your period.

The physical adjustments that accompany breastfeeding usually have little or no effect on breastfeeding success. With careful breastfeeding management, nursing can be continued during the treatment of routine problems, and more serious complications can be avoided entirely, allowing you and your baby to enjoy the benefits of breastfeeding for many months.

AT A GLANCE

Making Physical Adjustments to Childbirth and Breastfeeding

Body Changes After Birth

- Rest is vital if you are to recover quickly from childbirth and establish a good milk supply.
- Breastfeeding helps the uterus return to its prepregnant size quickly.
- Returning to your prepregnant shape will take many months.
- Lactating breasts are normally lumpy. If you suspect problems, however, consult your doctor.

Leaking

- Leaking is normal, especially before your milk supply has adjusted to your baby's demands.
- To minimize leaking, nurse frequently, keep your breasts empty, and avoid practices that produce excessive nipple stimulation.
- To control leaking, put temporary pressure on your breasts and wear breast pads.

Plugged Ducts

- To avoid plugged ducts, keep your breasts empty, vary nursing positions, and avoid placing continuous pressure on your breasts.
- To clear a plugged duct, nurse frequently, offer the affected breast first, position the baby so that his chin points toward the plug, massage your breasts to move the plug downwards, and apply moist heat.

Breast Infections

- A breast infection can be caused by fatigue, an irregular nursing pattern, an untreated plugged duct, or an illness spread by a family member.

- Symptoms of a breast infection include red, hot, tender areas of the breast, and flu-like symptoms such as chills, fever, aches, and fatigue.
- Treat breast infections with warm moist compresses, frequent nursings that keep the breast empty, total bed rest, and—if necessary— an antibiotic prescribed by your doctor.
- Breastfeeding usually can and should be continued during the treatment of a breast infection.

Menstruation

- Menstruation can return as early as 6 weeks postpartum, but might not occur until the baby weans.
- It is perfectly safe to nurse while menstruating.
- You may become fertile before the onset of menstruation. Take precautions!

9

Breastfeeding Your Baby at Home

Because hospital procedure may restrict your involvement with your baby, you will probably find that breastfeeding becomes much more pleasurable and easy to manage once you and your baby are finally able to settle into your daily routine at home. As your baby grows, you will observe changes in his nursing pattern, as well as other developmental factors related to breastfeeding. It is important to keep in mind that babies differ in their behavior, and that your baby will be unique in his own growth pattern and behavioral responses.

YOUR BABY'S NURSING BEHAVIOR

Once you are home with your baby, continue to respond to his needs by nursing when he wishes. Be aware that babies nurse for reasons other than hunger. Nursing has a calming effect and helps to soothe a baby who is upset or uncomfortable. It also fulfills a baby's sucking need, a requirement that varies among babies. By satisfying your baby's sucking need, you will enhance his emotional development and well-being.

Your baby's demands will be greatest during the first three months, and will decline as he matures. If you must be away from your baby for regular periods, you can compensate by responding to your baby during the times you are together. He may nurse frequently to make up for the absence. When possible, allow him to set the pace.

Increased Feedings

Once in a while, you may notice that your baby wants to nurse more frequently than he did previously. In fact, he may seem to nurse almost constantly for a day or two. Your initial reaction may be to worry that your milk supply is low and that your baby is hungry and unsatisfied. Actually your baby will probably be experiencing a spurt in his growth, and his frequent nursings will be a healthy response to his increased need for milk.

The increase in nipple stimulation caused by these additional feedings will signal your body to produce more milk. After a day or two, you should be making enough milk to satisfy his increased appetite, and your baby will probably return to his former nursing schedule. If you respond to your baby's natural instincts and do not interfere with this normal means of increasing milk production, you will continue to meet your baby's needs.

The following list will provide you with an approximate timetable of these intensive nursing times. Of course, your baby's individual growth pattern will establish his own periods of increased nursings. Many mothers who nurse their babies on a need-feed schedule, paying no attention to the clock or to the number of feedings in a day, are unaware of these changes in frequency.

Typical Times for Increased Feedings

The first days home. This is actually your baby's way of establishing his own nursing schedule, as opposed to the one he was on in the hospital. More frequent nursings at this time may also be his response to the change in environment, and may indicate a need for comfort rather than a need for food. If you were able to nurse directly after birth and were allowed to set your own need-feed schedule immediately, you may not notice a change in frequency at this time.

The ten-to-fourteen-day growth spurt. In addition to more frequent feedings, you may notice that the fullness in your breasts diminishes at this time. Don't misinterpret this change in breast size as an indication that your milk supply is low. You are merely losing the extra blood volume that accompanied pregnancy and the initial production of milk.

The four-to-six-week growth spurt. By this time, you may be resuming social and physical activities. Watch for signs that you are overdoing and, in turn, diminishing your milk supply. If your baby is unusually fussy for longer than a few days, you may have to decrease your activity level.

The three-month and six-month growth spurts. Don't misinterpret your baby's more frequent feedings at these times as an indication that he is not satisfied by a diet of breast milk alone, and is ready for solid foods. Respond to these growth spurts in the same way you reacted to others—by nursing whenever your baby is hungry. However, if increased feedings at six months or older do not satisfy your baby, he may be ready for solid foods. Chapter 12 provides guidelines for introducing solid foods into your baby's diet.

Other times. At times, your baby may nurse more frequently in response to illness, overstimulation, emotional distress, or physical discomfort. Again, remember that babies nurse for security and comfort as well as nourishment, and that your baby will be soothed by these additional nursings. For more information on breastfeeding your baby when he is ill, refer to page 205.

When Babies Prefer One Breast

Some babies prefer one breast and refuse to nurse from the other. Each breast is unique in size and shape, and your baby may respond to the differences between your breasts by showing a preference for one. Other factors, too, may cause your baby to develop a preference for one breast. If you tend to hold your baby in the same position at every feeding, you may transmit your own right- or left-handed preference to your baby. A stronger scent of deodorant or body lotion could also cause the rejection of one breast. A plugged duct, which can alter the taste or flow of milk in the affected breast, may also influence your baby's choice.

If your baby exhibits a breast preference, begin each feeding with the breast he favors. Your baby may be more willing to nurse from the opposite breast after he has established letdown and does not have to suck as hard. Pre-expressing drops of milk from the other breast may make it more appealing. Perhaps your baby can be fooled into thinking he is nursing from the preferred breast by being held in either the football or transverse position, with his body turned in the direction that is most familiar to him when he nurses on the preferred side. (See page 74 for illustrations of these nursing positions.)

YOUR BABY'S WEIGHT

When doctors examine a baby's weight-gain pattern, they usually rely on weight charts developed by formula companies as their standard of comparison. Many babies, whether fed breast milk or formula, generally lose between 5 and 10 percent of their birth weight during the first week of life. Following this initial weight loss, breast-fed babies whose feedings are restricted may exhibit a slower weight gain in the early weeks than formula-fed babies. During the second week after birth, their weight usually levels off. By the third week, they begin gaining. By the end of three weeks, they are usually close to birth weight. When feedings are unrestricted, however, the weight-gain pattern during the first three weeks of life may be very similar to that of formula-fed babies.

For the first four to five months, your baby will gain on the average of four to seven ounces a week. Again, keep in mind that these figures describe the average breast-fed baby; your baby may gain somewhat less or more and still be perfectly healthy. Some babies gain as much as one pound a week during the first few months, after which their weight-gain pattern begins to taper off. Take into account your own family's growth patterns. For instance, if you and your baby's father are of small stature, you can expect your baby's weight gain to be below the average. Most important is a steady, consistent pattern of growth.

When a Baby Appears to Gain Too Much Weight

Studies show that fat cells produced during infancy may cause obesity in later life. This concerns many parents, who worry that their babies may be gaining too much weight. Generally, a breast-fed baby who is allowed to establish his own feeding schedule will not be overfed. While it is normal for an infant to gain one to one and a half pounds per month for the first four to five months, this rapid gain should not continue beyond that time. Keep in mind that weight varies dramatically from one family to another, and that a steady gain of one pound a week may be perfectly normal for your baby during the first few months.

If you suspect that your baby is gaining weight too rapidly, review your nursing pattern to determine if you are encouraging your baby to nurse at times when he is not actually hungry. Some mothers too frequently rely on breastfeeding as a way of soothing their babies. If you feel this is the case, try other ways of calming your child. You may want to seek the advice of your doctor if you are concerned about excessive weight gain.

When a Baby Is Not Gaining Well

If you feel that your baby is not gaining weight at a safe rate, have him monitored closely by his doctor. In addition, you may wish to critically examine your breastfeeding practices. Make sure that your baby is positioned well at the breast and that he nurses long enough to receive the fatty hindmilk. Also, check the frequency of feedings and increase the number of nursings to at least eight per day. Discontinue the use of a pacifier, baby swing, and all other soothing techniques, replacing them with nursing as a means of comfort. By massaging the lower portion of your breast while you are nursing, you will increase the milk flow, and your baby will consequently receive a greater amount of milk at each feeding. (See page 213 for a description of breast massage.)

Review your own state of mind, personal habits, and activity level. Emotional stress can interfere with your letdown reflex, as can cigarette smoking and certain drugs. If your milk does not let down, your baby will be poorly nourished. Fatigue, birth control pills, and drugs such as antihistamines can also interfere with milk production, resulting in a low milk supply.

Poor weight gain is a common problem of placid babies. A placid baby may sleep as much as eighteen to twenty hours a day, and makes few demands for attention. He does not cry to let you know he is awake and hungry, and so he soon falls asleep again, remaining unfed. If you notice this type of behavior, monitor your baby closely, checking him at intervals of two or three hours to wake and feed him. A noisy device such as a bell, rattle, or other play toy placed in his crib may help you to hear him when he awakens. Most important, keep in mind that you cannot rely on a placid baby for cues that he is hungry; you must initiate feedings yourself.

Sometimes, babies with a low birth weight or a weak sucking reflex fail to gain weight well. This may be due to an inability to nurse for sufficiently long periods of time. To aid these babies in obtaining milk, initiate letdown by massaging the breast and hand expressing prior to feedings. Pre-expressing the foremilk will make the rich hindmilk immediately available for the baby's nourishment. Since the baby will tire easily during feedings, offer only one breast at each nursing, and feed him once every hour. Continued poor weight gain can result in a more serious condition, called **failure to thrive**, and should be monitored closely by the baby's doctor.

YOUR MILK SUPPLY

A common question asked by breastfeeding mothers is "How will I know if I have enough milk for my baby?" Your breasts will be so full when your milk first comes in that you will feel confident of a good milk supply. Once your baby has been nursing for a couple of weeks, however, you may notice that your breasts have lost most of their fullness, and think that you have also lost your milk. Again, remember that this loss of fullness in your breasts is normal and is not a sign of inadequate milk production.

There are a number of things you can watch for to determine if your baby is being well-nourished. Provided that your baby is receiving no supplements or water, one reliable indication of a plentiful milk supply is a pattern of at least six to eight soaked diapers a day. If you use suprerabsorbent disposable diapers, your baby will probably soak three to five diapers daily. The use of fewer diapers and the presence of consistently dark urine may mean that your baby is not getting enough milk.

Your baby is being well fed if he nurses six to ten times a day, is positioned correctly, and nurses long enough at the breast. Observe him to determine if he seems satisfied for several hours after feedings, with regular intervals of wakefulness and sleep. If your baby exhibits good skin tone, has fat creases in his arms and legs, outgrows his clothes frequently, and shows other signs of good health, you can feel confident that he is being well fed.

Increasing Your Milk Supply

If you suspect that your milk supply is low, you can take measures to increase it. Milk production is a direct result of nipple stimulation, so if you breastfeed more frequently—every one and a half to two hours—you will produce more milk. Again, make sure your baby nurses long enough on one breast before offering him the other one, so that he receives the high-calorie hindmilk.

You will need to get plenty of rest—no easy task with a busy work or social schedule! Cut down on activities as much as possible, and take your baby to bed with you to nurse while lying down. This will not only give you the rest you need, but will provide your baby with skin-to-skin contact, encouraging him to nurse more frequently.

Careful attention to your diet is important when trying to increase a low milk supply. Eat foods that are high in protein and the B vitamins: meat, fish, poultry, eggs, cheese, nuts, liver, and green leafy vegetables. Be sure to get enough calories by eating three well-balanced meals and two or three healthful snacks each day.

Managing Temporary Supplements

If your baby is failing to gain weight or is gaining weight very slowly, his doctor may prescribe formula supplements. Work closely with the doctor to ensure that breastfeeding remains your baby's primary source of nourishment. Nursings should become very frequent to increase your milk supply. Rather than letting your baby take all the formula he wants, offer specific amounts. Offering the formula in a nursing supplementer will allow you to supplement during nursing times and avoid bottles that could cause sucking confusion. If formula is offered at a separate time, use a dropper or cup.

When your baby's weight gain becomes satisfactory, you will be able to slowly decrease supplements as your own milk supply increases through more frequent nursings. If you are not using a nursing supplementer, breastfeed first and offer the formula afterwards. If you find that your baby is satisfied with nursing and does not want the formula, reduce the amount accordingly, eliminating a half an ounce per day, or even more if your baby is doing well.

Never dilute your baby's formula. If you find that he is satisfied with less formula, decrease the amount you give him, but not the strength. Try to have realistic expectations, and watch for small daily successes. It is not reasonable to try to wean your baby from supplements overnight, or even in two or three days. It will take time and patience.

YOUR BABY'S DIGESTIVE PATTERNS

Nursing mothers sometimes believe that all of their baby's body functions are related to breastfeeding. Some digestive patterns, such as loose stools, are acceptable variations associated with breastfeeding. Others, such as burping and spitting up, are common to all babies. All babies differ in their digestive patterns, whether they are nourished by breast milk or by infant formula. Resist the trap of blaming routine differences on the fact that you are breastfeeding. By familiarizing yourself with the body functions of a normal breast-fed baby and evaluating your baby's behavior in light of these patterns, you will avoid a great deal of unnecessary worry.

When Your Baby Spits Up

Your baby may spit up or dribble milk from his mouth quite often during his first months. He may even spit up several times during one feeding. As your baby's digestive system matures, this behavior will probably disappear. Frequent spitting up could be caused by overfeeding, an overactive letdown reflex, or gulping caused by excessive hunger. It could also result from mucus in your baby's stomach, which is common directly after birth and whenever your baby has a cold. Allergies to nicotine or cow's milk may also cause spitting up, necessitating adjustments in your diet or personal habits.

Because the stomach opens to the esophagus on the left side, you may be able to reduce your baby's spitting up by laying him on his right side for sleeping. Any air bubble that rises will then have less of a chance of being accompanied by milk. It may not be necessary to nurse your baby at both breasts during each feeding. If your baby seems to become overly full regularly, you can limit him to one breast at each feeding. Short, frequent nursings will also help your baby to avoid overfullness.

If you are concerned about the amount of milk being spit up, try to determine the actual quantity. Pour one tablespoon of water onto a cloth and observe how far it spreads. A little bit of liquid often looks like a great deal more when it spills. Normal spitting up is not a cause for concern. But if your baby often spits up more than a tablespoon of milk, or frequently vomits with great force, you should contact your doctor to rule out a more serious cause.

Your Baby's Bowel Habits

A breast-fed baby's bowel movements have a significantly looser consistency than those of a formula-fed baby, and the odor is much less unpleasant. The consistency will vary from one that is similar to toothpaste to one that is watery with curds. There may also be mucus present in the early days or at times when your baby has a cold. The color may be black, brown, green, or yellow. A dark color is most common during the first two to three days, when your baby is passing meconium.

Babies' bowel habits can differ greatly, as there is a wide range of normality. Most babies have at least one bowel movement daily in the early days. Some have a soiled diaper at every change! As he matures, your baby's bowel habits will change in terms of frequency and consistency, especially once solid foods have been introduced into his diet. While you can expect some variation, you should consult your doctor about any sudden changes in your baby's pattern.

Constipation is rare in breast-fed infants. Do not misinterpret your baby's straining to move his bowels as a sign of constipation; some degree of pushing is normal. Constipation is characterized by firm stools and a great deal of straining. While uncommon, it could occur as a result of something in your diet that passes through to the breast milk. Diarrhea, while also rare, is a frequent side effect when a baby or mother is being treated with an antibiotic.

WHEN YOUR BABY IS DISTRESSED

A baby's cries are not always a sign of hunger. Babies also cry to communicate feelings of discomfort or loneliness. Cries of pain, hunger, or the need for companionship all have different sounds. As you and your baby spend more time together, you will learn to distinguish between his different cries. If you find it difficult to determine whether your baby is hungry or is crying in response to some physical or emotional discomfort, try to remember when he last nursed. A baby usually cries from hunger one and a half to two hours after a good feeding.

And, how do you know if your baby has had a good feeding, to rule out hunger as the cause of his crying? First, make sure you are positioning him well at the breast. If not, he may nurse for an extended time but not receive sufficient nourishment. Also, make sure he has sucked long enough at the breast to get the high-calorie hindmilk.

If you feel confident that your baby has had a good feeding, you can then explore reasons other than hunger for his discomfort. He may find the sensation of a full stomach uncomfortable. He may need to burp. He may have to pass gas or a large bowel movement. These issues will be resolved as he matures.

A baby who cries at the breast and refuses to nurse presents quite a challenge. You can usually calm an older baby by putting him to breast. A newborn, however, will be contented at the breast only if he is hungry. If you try to nurse him when he is not hungry, he may cry even harder!

When your baby is fussy and cannot be comforted by nursing, take heart! There are other ways to soothe him. Cuddle him at the breast for the comfort of skin-to-skin contact. If he is willing, place your index finger in his mouth with the nail side down against his tongue so that he can suck on it.

Some form of artificial pacifier has been around probably as long as rubber bottle nipples. But, pacifiers can create problems for breastfeeding babies, and so should be avoided.

When an artificial nipple is placed in a breast-fed baby's mouth, his instinct will be to thrust his tongue upwards, mirroring his actions at the breast. However, this action will push the artificial nipple out of the baby's mouth. If the baby is encouraged to suck on the pacifier, he will become confused by the different sucking action required to keep it in his mouth. Mothers find their babies are usually comforted quite easily by sucking on their own fists or their mother's finger.

More techniques for comforting your baby appear on page 70. Remember that by meeting your baby's needs in infancy, you are fostering a sense of security and trust.

The Colicky Baby

Sometimes a baby's cries become so intense that special measures are needed to soothe him. If your baby appears to be in severe discomfort most of the time, has a piercing cry, and draws his legs up sharply to his abdomen or becomes rigid and arches his back, he may have colic. His continuous crying will cause him to swallow air and develop more gas, which will further aggravate his discomfort.

It is not clearly understood what causes colic. Some experts think that it is associated with an immature digestive system or with allergies. Other experts believe that it is the result of an overly sensitive nervous system, which could cause the baby to respond with discomfort to most stimuli. The fact that colic symptoms usually disappear by the time the baby reaches three to six months of age seems to support the theory that it is related to an immaturity of the baby's system.

Relieving Your Baby's Discomfort

You can do a number of things to dramatically reduce the duration and intensity of your baby's colic symptoms. Massaging your baby with a firm touch will provide him with comforting skin-to-skin contact. In fact, regular massages may relieve your baby's colic in as little as one or two weeks. Another effective soothing technique is swaddling, which comforts the baby by restricting his movements. To help your baby release tension and pass gas, keep him warm by covering him with sweaters or blankets, or by placing a hot water bottle over his stomach. Repeatedly folding his legs onto his stomach will also help your baby to pass gas.

Other techniques that are recommended for soothing a colicky baby are rocking, swinging, walking, and riding in a car, all of which provide a constant, steady motion. Steady, continuous sounds such as the noise of a vacuum cleaner, humming, singing, or a tape recording of your own heartbeat may provide comfort, too. It has also been reported that a baby stops crying when he hears a recording of his own cry. If the colic is severe, your doctor may prescribe medication to relieve your baby's discomfort.

A colicky baby should receive short, frequent feedings, so that his stomach does not become too full at any one time. He will also need to be burped often to release the gas bubbles caused by tension and crying. All potential allergens should be removed from his diet, including supplements of vitamins, fluoride, and iron. To avoid passing allergens through your milk, monitor your own food intake as well. In a 1983 study, the colic symptoms of one third of a group of breast-fed infants disappeared in one to three days when the infants' mothers were put on a diet that was free of cow's milk.[1] This suggests that your avoidance of cow's milk and other dairy products could reduce or eliminate your baby's colic symptoms. If you decide to remove dairy products from your diet, be sure to substitute other forms of calcium and protein so that your nutritional needs will continue to be satisfied.

Your Own State of Mind

While your primary concern will be the alleviation of your baby's discomfort, your own distress should not be minimized. It is understandable that you may become frustrated, tired, and upset when caring for a baby who constantly cries with pain. Occasionally, you will need some relief from caring for your baby. In fact, he may pick up on your own tension, and may be comforted more easily when someone else holds him. Both of you might benefit from some time spent away from each other.

Keeping a written record of your baby's periods of sleep, fussiness, and feedings will help you to get a clear picture of his condition. You may find that the fussiness is not as constant as you had perceived. Take heart in knowing that the vast majority of colicky babies develop into calm, good-natured children.

YOUR BABY'S SLEEPING PATTERN

Many parents wonder if their baby's sleeping pattern is affected by breastfeeding. Specifically, they question whether breastfeeding is the cause of their baby's inability to sleep through the night. As is true of all other infant behavior, sleeping habits vary dramatically among babies. Some begin sleeping for long periods at night when they are only a few days old, while others do not sleep through the night until after their first birthday. A number of factors—including development, personality, environment, and hunger—will have an influence on your baby's sleeping schedule.

Changing Needs for Sleep

Your baby will begin sleeping for longer periods as his central nervous system becomes more mature. On the average, babies begin sleeping for a span of five or six hours at about three months of age. Hopefully, this long sleeping period will be at night, and not during the day!

Personality can also be a factor. Some babies like to go to sleep early and awaken early, while others prefer going to sleep late and rising late in the morning. Not too different from adults! Many babies go through a period of separation anxiety at about five to eight months of age. They may awaken frequently during the night and, finding themselves alone, have difficulty returning to sleep. Discomfort from teething, colds, and earaches can also affect your baby's sleep.

Encouraging Sleep

Anything that affects your baby's senses of touch, sight, hearing, or smell can have an impact on his sleeping pattern. If he is allowed to become overly tired or stimulated, he may have difficulty settling down. Watch for signs that your baby is sleepy, and plan quiet, soothing activities before bedtime. The temperature of your baby's bedroom and bedding should be comfortably warm, but not hot. Lambskin and flannel sheets have been found effective in providing added warmth and comfort. If the humidity in the room is too low, your baby may have difficulty breathing. This can be remedied with the use of a cool air vaporizer.

You can encourage your baby to sleep longer at night by nursing him directly before you go to bed. If you find that he is sleeping for longer periods during the day, rather than at night, try waking him every three hours during the day to nurse. You should be able to alter his schedule within a few days.

When Your Baby Wakes From Hunger

Breast milk is digested easily and quickly. It seems reasonable, therefore, that a breast-fed baby would be hungry more often than a formula-fed baby, and would awaken periodically at night for feedings. However, the number of nighttime feedings for breast-fed and formula-fed babies seems fairly comparable, while frequent nursings are most prevalent during the day.

When your baby does awaken to nurse at night, try to limit stimulation so that he will be able to fall back to sleep more easily. Keep him warm, and keep a night light in his room so that you won't have to turn on any bright lights. Change his diaper before nursing him on the second breast so that he can go to sleep as soon as the feeding is over. By double diapering your baby before putting him to bed, you may be able to avoid diaper changes during the night.

If daytime responsibilities frequently take you away from home, your baby may awaken during the night to enjoy the nursings and skin contact that were missed during your absence. These night feedings can be very special, enabling you and your baby to enjoy unhurried, uninterrupted time together.

Night feedings need not rob you of your own rest. Bring your baby to bed with you, and nurse lying down. Don't hesitate to keep your baby in bed for the entire night. The warmth and familiar smell of your body will comfort him. If you are afraid that your baby will fall off the bed, place a mattress on the floor or push your bed next to the wall. Many mothers worry that they may roll over and smother the baby, but this is unlikely. You will be aware, even if only subconsciously, that your baby is with you.

When Your Baby Begins to Sleep Through the Night

When your baby first begins sleeping through the night—and you thought it would never happen!—you may experience some initial discomfort from fullness in your breasts. Your body, unable to anticipate that your baby would begin sleeping for such a long period, will continue to produce milk for night feedings. When you awaken in the morning, your breasts may be full from the extra milk. You may even be awakened by the discomfort of fullness in the middle of the night.

To avoid overly full breasts, try nursing your baby directly before you go to bed. This may require that you awaken him to nurse, but he will fall back to sleep easily after his stomach is full. You might also awaken him to nurse as soon as you rise in the morning, or hand express your milk to relieve the pressure until he awakens on his own for a feeding. If you are terribly uncomfortable during the night, you may, again, choose to awaken your baby to nurse. Be assured that this breast fullness will not last long. Once your baby has been sleeping through the night for a few days, your body will respond accordingly by decreasing milk production during the night hours.

The early weeks at home with your baby will be a time of wonderment and joy—a time when you and your baby get to know each other, and you become acquainted with all of your baby's special qualities and needs. Soon you will be past the initial period of adjustment, and will have a clear understanding of your baby's behavior. With this understanding will come an increased confidence in your ability as a mother and, in turn, an increased enjoyment of the nursing relationship.

AT A GLANCE

Breastfeeding Your Baby at Home

Baby's Nursing Behavior

- Babies nurse for comfort and security as well as nourishment.
- Growth spurts occur at fairly predictable times and cause a baby nurse more frequently for a day or two.
- Don't nurse your baby every time he cries; learn to distinguish between different cries, and first try other means of comfort.
- Use a pacifier wisely; it is an aid in satisfying sucking needs, not a substitute for mothering or adequate feedings.
- Babies sometimes prefer one breast over the other. Measures can be taken to encourage your baby to nurse from both breasts.
- Small amounts of spitting up are normal, and should not cause concern.

Baby's Weight Gain

- Usually, breast-fed babies lose weight during the first week and turn to their birth weight by the end of the third week.
- Weight-gain patterns vary dramatically, depending on family stature and other factors.
- Normal weight gain is about 4 to 7 ounces per week for the first 4 to 5 months.
- If your baby does not gain well, consult his doctor and take measures to build your milk supply and increase feedings.
- If your baby gains weight too rapidly, review your breastfeeding management and decrease feedings if necessary.
- If your baby is placid and fails to cry when hungry, monitor him closely and initiate feedings yourself.

Your Milk Supply

- 6 to 8 soaked diapers daily indicate a good milk supply.
- A pleasant disposition and regular intervals of wakefulness and sleep are signs of a well-nourished baby.
- A steady pattern of weight gain and growth, healthy skin tone,

and fat creases in your baby's arms and legs are all signs of normal growth.

- Nurse 6 to 10 times a day to maintain your milk supply.
- To increase your milk supply, nurse more frequently, get plenty of rest, eat a well-balanced diet, and decrease formula supplements.

Bowel Habits

- The stool consistency of a breast-fed baby is normally loose, varying from that of toothpaste to that of liquid with curds.
- Stool color ranges from black to light yellow.
- The frequency of bowel movements varies, ranging from one after every feeding to one a day in the early days.

Crying and Colic

- Colic symptoms include severe discomfort, piercing cries, sharp gas pains, the drawing up of legs, and rigidity of the body.
- Short, frequent feedings will prevent the overfullness that can aggravate colic.
- Avoid allergens in your diet that can pass through to your milk. Cow's milk, especially, should be avoided in the event of colic.
- Several techniques can be used to soothe a colicky baby, including massage, continuous motion or sound, warmth, and swaddling.
- Colic symptoms usually disappear in 3 to 6 months.
- If colic persists, obtain a prescribed medication from your baby's doctor.

Sleeping Patterns

- Sleeping patterns are affected by environment, infant development, nutrition, and individual personality, but not by feeding methods.
- Babies begin to sleep through the night at widely different ages.

10

Adjusting to Your New Family

Relationships with family members may take on new dimensions with the birth of your baby. You and your mate will gradually have to redefine some aspects of your relationship as a couple to accommodate parenthood. No longer will the two of you be totally absorbed in each other's needs. Your baby will become the focus of your attention, the center of your life. There will be times when you must put aside your individual interests in order to respond to the immediate needs of your baby.

When a second or third baby is born, additional adjustments will be necessary as you make room for each new family member. Older children will require more of your time and understanding as they adjust to a new sibling, and these adjustments may become more marked when you choose to breastfeed your baby. Even your relationship with your own parents may change as they learn to view you as a new parent, with all the responsibilities and decisions that accompany that role.

UNDERSTANDING YOUR EMOTIONS

While some women adjust to the arrival of a new baby easily, others experience depression and temporary difficulties. Emotional mood swings are common in the early weeks after delivery. It may help to understand that your body goes through a temporary hormonal imbalance after you give birth, and that this imbalance can significantly affect your emotions. If you were involved in a career or social activities before your baby was born, you may find it difficult to adjust to being at home. Life may seem lonely and intellectually boring with no adult contact—especially without other new mothers with whom you can share your feelings and experiences. You may wish to get in touch with a local support group for new parents or breastfeeding women. Speaking to other mothers who are going through the same adjustments may help you to regain your perspective.

Perhaps you even feel unprepared to care for your baby. Mothering is a learned skill, and this skill will grow as you practice, experiment, observe your baby, and educate yourself. Try to develop realistic expectations. The "super mom" myth is just that—a myth.

A healthy diet will be essential to your adjustment. Be especially careful to eat a nutritious breakfast so that your blood sugar level remains constant. An erratic blood sugar level can cause both your emotions and your energy to fluctuate. Physical exercise, too, will enhance your feeling of well-being. Aerobic exercise is particularly beneficial, as it improves circulation. Take care to get adequate rest, as fatigue will tax both your body and your mind.

MAKING SEXUAL ADJUSTMENTS

Re-establishing sexual relations with your mate is one of many steps that will lead to a complete adjustment to your new role. This renewal of your relationship, however, may be complicated by ambivalent or confused emotions. Are you feeling a bit apprehensive and awkward as you try to resume your sexual relationship? Although eager to be alone with your partner, by bedtime are you too exhausted to do anything but sleep? While you usually enjoy the closeness of making love, at times do you feel that you receive so much love and emotional gratification from your nursing baby that you don't need affection from your mate?

If you experience any of these emotions, be assured that you share them with many other new mothers. The need to adapt to a renewed sex life is common to many couples. It is crucial that you communicate openly with each other about your feelings and allow each other the time to make this important adjustment.

Resuming Intercourse

Most health professionals recommend waiting until after the six-week gynecologic checkup before resuming sex. Your sexual desire and responses may take several months to return, and you may need time to renew your enthusiasm. Studies show, however, that most women choose to resume intercourse earlier than six weeks postpartum, and that no detrimental effects have been demonstrated even at two weeks after delivery.[1] Until you resume relations, you and your mate can rekindle tenderness by cuddling and holding each other.

Many breastfeeding women believe that they should avoid fondling and other forms of foreplay that involve their breasts. If this concerns you, you can cleanse your breasts before nursing; be aware, though, that there is no danger to your baby. Breast sensitivity may be altered for a time due to stimulation received during nursing. You may find that your breasts are either overly sensitive or unresponsive to foreplay. Both of these reactions are perfectly normal and will pass with time.

Because the hormones associated with breastfeeding will cause a decrease in vaginal lubrication, you may wish to use a product such as K-Y Jelly artificial lubricant. When orgasm is reached during lovemaking, oxytocin is released, which may cause your milk to let down, resulting in leaking. To remedy this, empty your breasts through nursing or manual expression before you have intercourse, and keep a towel handy for any leakage that does occur. You may also want to adjust your position during lovemaking to avoid placing pressure on your breasts.

The Sensuality of Nursing

It is perfectly normal to experience some sexual arousal while nursing. This sensation disturbs some women, who feel that such a sexual response is inappropriate. However, nursing provides a very warm, intimate bond between a mother and her baby, and it is natural to encounter sensual enjoyment when nursing your baby.

CHOOSING A METHOD OF BIRTH CONTROL

There are many factors you may want to consider when choosing a reliable method of contraception. Naturally, your choice must be one that is compatible with breastfeeding. Since many women use birth control pills as a contraceptive prior to pregnancy, and are familiar with them, they may consider using them after delivery. However, it has been shown that the estrogen in the pill may decrease milk production.[2] More important, the long-term effects of the pill on infants are not fully known. Therefore, *nursing mothers should not use high-estrogen birth control pills.*

Informative books, pamphlets, leaflets, and personal counseling are available through Planned Parenthood. You and your mate may also wish to discuss birth control issues with your health care provider. Some considerations are:

- Religious or ethical feelings about birth control.
- Effectiveness of the method chosen.
- Responsibility for birth control. Can it be used with alternative methods? Is the responsibility solely the woman's?
- Convenience. Will you remember to use it?
  Will you want to use it?
- Spontaneity.
- Expense.
- Feelings about the use of foreign objects.
- Messiness.
- Allergic reactions to ingredients, and other health considerations.

Finding a Method That's Compatible With Breastfeeding

Several birth control options are open to nursing mothers. They are presented below, in order of effectiveness. Contact your doctor for more detailed information on specific methods.

Sterilization. This involves either a vasectomy for the male or tubal ligation for the female. Ducts carrying sperm or the egg are tied and cut surgically. Sterilization is reported to be almost 100 percent effective.

Foam and condom. A rubber device shaped to fit over the penis is used to prevent sperm from entering the vagina, while a spermicidal foam is placed in the vagina. This combination is reported to be almost 100 percent effective.

Intrauterine device (IUD). A piece of plastic with nylon or copper threads attached is placed in the uterus. Although reported to be 95 to 99 percent effective, its safety is now being questioned, and it is contraindicated for nursing mothers because of the increased risk of uterine perforation.

Diaphragm. A rubber cup is placed in the vagina to form a barrier between the uterus and the sperm, while a spermicidal jelly or cream is used to kill the sperm. This method is reported to be about 97 percent effective.

Cervical cap. A small barrier-type device is filled with a spermicidal jelly or cream and placed over the cervix. Its reliability is equal to that of the diaphragm. Currently, the device is available only through research studies conducted by health clinics in most major cities. Approval by the Federal Drug Administration is pending, but five years of research have shown no detrimental effects, and researchers consider it to be a safe and effective contraceptive.

Total natural family planning. Total natural family planning, which is also referred to as periodic abstinence, involves charting the basal body temperature, checking vaginal secretions, and keeping a careful calendar record of menstrual periods in order to predict fertile days and avoid intercourse at that time. It is reported to be 90 to 97 percent effective. Total natural family planning should not he confused with the calendar rhythm method, in which fertile days are computed solely on the basis of calendar records. The calendar method, which has a low rate of effectiveness, cannot be relied upon to prevent pregnancy.

Jellies, foams, and creams. Spermicidal agents are inserted directly into the vagina to destroy sperm and act as a physical barrier between sperm and the uterus. This method is reported to be 90 to 97 percent effective.

Sponge. A disposable soft polyurethane material that is permeated with a spermicide is placed in the vagina to kill sperm and act as a barrier. It is reported to remain effective for 24 hours. Caution should be used with this product, as it can cause toxic shock syndrome if not used according to the manufacturer's directions. It is reported to be 86 percent effective.

Relying on Breastfeeding as a Contraceptive

If you are breastfeeding and not menstruating, you cannot become pregnant, right? Wrong! Many women become fertile before the onset of their first menstrual periods. Do not assume that you are infertile merely because you are not menstruating.

It is true that ovulation is inhibited by the high levels of prolactin produced by breastfeeding. However, frequent nursings are necessary to maintain a high prolactin level; if frequency decreases, so will the level of prolactin. Nursing your baby often, for a prolonged period of time and with very little supplementation of other foods, will help you to remain infertile. Help is the key word; breastfeeding should be regarded as an aid to child spacing rather than a means of preventing pregnancy.

When using breastfeeding as a form of contraception, you should be alert to any changes in your baby's nursing pattern. The delicate balance of hormones can fluctuate because of missed feedings, the introduction of supplements or solid foods, the elimination of night feedings, or even the use of a pacifier. Watch for signs that ovulation is returning, such as increased vaginal secretions, and always use a back-up method of birth control if you do not wish to risk pregnancy.

ADJUSTING TO FATHERHOOD

New fathers of breastfeeding babies often feel left out, and perhaps even a little envious of the relationship enjoyed by the mother and baby. A father wants to take part in his baby's care. He also has his own needs for attention and affection. By spending special time alone with your mate, you will help your relationship remain warm and affectionate. Either arrange for a relative or friend to care for your baby, or take advantage of those times when your baby is asleep.

Let your mate know that you have confidence in his ability to care for your baby. He may not do things in the same way you would, and will probably be a little awkward and unsure of himself in the beginning (new mothers don't have a corner on that market!). He will respond much better to support and encouragement than he will to hovering or criticism. If the undershirt is on backwards or the diaper is too loose, your baby won't know or care!

His Role With the Baby

Although breastfeeding will prevent your partner from being involved in feedings during the early months, there are many ways in which he can get to know your baby. Soon after birth, he can learn the skills needed for baby care. When your baby is fussy, he can soothe him by walking, rocking, singing, and cooing. He can bathe, burp, diaper, and play with your baby. When the baby is old enough to receive a bottle, your mate can feed him. Night feedings will be made easier for you if he brings the baby to you, enabling you to remain in bed. All of this early involvement will help to prepare your mate for even greater interaction and enjoyment once your baby grows older and more responsive.

His Role as Your Helpmate

Your mate's patience, understanding, and concern will help to make breastfeeding and parenting more enjoyable for both of you. Since you will need rest during the early days, he can help with household tasks and relax his own standards of cleanliness and order. He can discourage visitors who stay too long or make you uncomfortable, and can defend your choice of breastfeeding when faced with those who are critical or unaccepting. A supportive mate can be your best line of defense and an indispensable source of emotional support.

SIBLING ADJUSTMENT

If you have other young children at home, you can prepare them for the birth of your new baby by educating them about pregnancy and birth. Read books together, look at the family's baby pictures, and discuss how babies change as they grow. Talk about what the new baby will do and need once he is home, explaining that newborns eat and sleep most of the time, with very short periods of wakefulness. Include your older child in preparations for the new baby. If your child's sleeping arrangements must be changed to accommodate the new baby, you may want to make the change early enough to allow him time to adjust.

Planning Ahead

Several weeks before you go to the hospital, prepare your child for the separation. Tell him where you will be, why you are going, what you will do, and how long you will be away. You may wish to visit the hospital with your child to acquaint him with the surroundings. Together, you can make a booklet of pictures that show the hospital, the arrival of the baby at your home, and ways of caring for a newborn.

Your child will feel more secure if he knows, well in advance, who will care for him in your absence. He will be most comfortable if he can remain in your home. If this is not possible, try to arrange for him to stay with someone who is familiar and close to him. Visiting this friend or relative with your child ahead of time will help to pave the way for a smooth transition.

If you plan to have your child attend the birth, be sure that he will know what to expect. Tailor your preparations to his age and maturity. Find a book at the public library or a local bookstore that explains and illustrates the birth process. Discuss your own birth plans, and answer his questions. Prior education will help to avoid unpleasant or frightening surprises that could result from his not knowing what is normal during labor and delivery. Arrange for another adult to care for your child while the birth is taking place—someone who can reassure him and explain what is happening.

After Your Baby Is Born

If you will be separated from your family directly after birth, you can keep in touch with your child by telephone and through pictures and notes. Try to arrange for your child to visit you and your new baby during your stay; many hospitals will at least allow a visit with the mother. When you first return home with your new baby, hand him to another family member so you can give your undivided attention to your older child, renewing contact and expressing your love and affection.

As you and the new baby settle in, let each child spend some time with him, looking at, touching, and holding him. In the days that follow, try to set aside a special time every day for each child. This will reassure each one that he is just as important to you as he was before the new baby arrived.

Mixed Reviews

Your patience and understanding will be crucial during this period of transition. While children often adjust comfortably to a new baby, be aware that there could be some difficult times. You may be faced with whining, baby talk, bedwetting, waking at night, clinging, and perhaps even hostile actions toward you or your new baby. Many children have mixed feelings about a new baby—loving him but not wanting to share you with him . . . loving you but acting angry and sullen. Accept your child's feelings, and encourage his involvement with the baby.

Your child's role in the family will be redefined and expanded. Show him how much fun it can be to play with and help care for a little baby. Talk about his own infancy, and the changes and growth that have taken place since then. He will be able to assume new responsibilities now that he is no longer a "baby." He won't always need someone to help him, because he is growing up and can do things for himself. Show him that he is important, and help him feel special in new ways. Encourage him to enjoy his new independence and self-reliance.

Sharing in Nursings

Many times, an older child wants to share in the growing closeness he sees between his mother and the new baby. By nursing your baby on the bed, couch, or floor, there will be room for all. To help you share nursings with your older child, you may wish to plan activities such as reading, playing a special game, or listening to records.

Your older child may ask to nurse and, if offered the breast, may giggle and not follow through. Your acceptance of his desire to try will show him that you still love him, and he will be reassured by your awareness of his needs and your willingness to comply. Although such a renewed interest in breastfeeding is usually temporary, some children continue requesting to nurse for some time. Often, they simply wish to taste the milk, and can be satisfied by drinking some out of a cup or spoon.

Adolescent Adjustment

The reactions of those children who are beyond the preschool years should also be considered. Young teens may be acutely embarrassed by the thought or sight of their mother using her breasts to feed a young baby. Adolescents will probably be exploring their own sexuality, and may be uncomfortable viewing their parents in sexual terms. Reactions may vary, especially between male and female adolescents, regarding the appropriate function of the breast.

You can help your child learn to view breastfeeding as a means of nurturing. Giving him an opportunity to watch you nurse may satisfy his curiosity and eliminate the uneasiness that results from a lack of familiarity with breastfeeding. Keep the lines of communication open so that your child will feel free to discuss the causes of his embarrassment or discomfort. You may also wish to consider your older child when choosing the time and location of feedings. If, for instance, you sense that he is embarrassed when feedings take place while his friends are visiting your home, you can avoid nursing in their presence.

WHEN OTHERS ARE UNSUPPORTIVE

You will be among the fortunate minority if you go through your entire nursing experience without receiving some degree of opposition. People who express displeasure with breastfeeding often do so because they do not understand it. Many times, educating them about the mechanics of breastfeeding and the needs of a breastfeeding baby will improve their attitudes. There are always some people, however, who are unrelenting in their comments and criticism. You may hear remarks such as:

- How long do you plan to nurse?
- Does he want to nurse again so soon?
- Maybe your milk isn't rich enough.
- Maybe you don't have enough milk.
- Are you still nursing?
- Isn't he too old to nurse?

Use your judgment in deciding how to respond to such remarks. Humor or a polite explanation may prove useful. There are times, however, when it is best to simply ignore the statement. You may need to avoid unsupportive people as much as possible and learn to turn a deaf ear to their comments.

When Your Mate's Support Wanes

When those who are important to you make unsupportive comments, it may be difficult for you to cope. To totally enjoy and feel comfortable about breastfeeding, you will need the support and encouragement of those close to you. If your mate expresses concern that your baby will become too dependent, give him reading material about the physical and emotional benefits your baby is receiving from breastfeeding. Assure him that satisfying your baby's emotional needs during infancy will encourage independence later. If your mate appears to be jealous or unhappy about the amount of time you must spend feeding your baby, make an extra effort to plan special times alone with him. Talk openly with him about his feelings, and let him know how important his support is to you.

If your mate's support seems to wane as your baby grows older, emphasize the benefits of breastfeeding a child throughout his development. A father's apparent opposition may actually be concern for the health and well-being of his mate or baby. He may merely need reassurance that you are both enjoying and benefiting from nursing. See Chapter 11 for more information on breastfeeding an older baby.

Mothers and Mothers-in-Law

If your mother or your mother-in-law expresses concern or apprehension about your breastfeeding, don't feel alone! Many women who had babies twenty to forty years ago were unable to breastfeed successfully. Breastfeeding was not popular at that time and was discouraged by many physicians. For those who wanted to breastfeed, there was a lack of support and helpful information.

Your mother may be concerned about you and your baby, and may want to shelter you from disappointment or failure. Perhaps she does not understand the normal nursing pattern, and worries that frequent feedings indicate a low milk supply. Try to accept her feelings and her point of view while helping her to understand your baby's needs and letting her know that her support is important to you.

Your Health Care Provider

At times, your health care provider may give you advice that you feel could compromise your breastfeeding. Tell him how important breastfeeding is to you and demonstrate your willingness to do whatever is necessary to continue. If you question a recommended procedure, find out—in a tactful manner—why the advice was given, and work together as a health care team to explore alternatives.

Before your medical appointment, prepare a list of specific questions. Health professionals are usually receptive to patients who present their concerns in a well-thought-out and confident fashion. If your concerns remain unresolved, however, you may wish to obtain a second opinion from another health provider.

You can enjoy successful breastfeeding despite the presence of unsupportive people. Apparent opposition can be turned around if you patiently educate those who do not understand your special needs. The process of redefining relationships may be both challenging and rewarding as you, your mate, and other family members learn to view one another in new ways and to share in the excitement of a new life.

AT A GLANCE

Adusting to Your New Family

Sexuality

- The need for sexual adjustment is common. You and your mate should share your feelings and allow each other time to adapt.
- Hormones may cause vaginal dryness. The use of an artificial lubricant will ease the discomfort caused by this dryness.
- Feelings of sexual arousal while breastfeeding are normal.

Contraception

- You may become fertile before the onset of menstruation; take precautions!
- Do not use high-estrogen birth control pills while breastfeeding; review alternatives.
- Although breastfeeding can be considered an aid to child spacing, you should always use a back-up method of birth control.

Your Emotional Adjustment

- Emotional mood swings are common in the early weeks after delivery.
- It is normal to feel unsure about your ability to care for your new baby. Be assured that your child care skills will grow with time and experience.
- Contact with other new mothers—possibly through a local breastfeeding group—may provide you with the emotional support that you need.

Family and Friends

- Give support and encouragement to the baby's father regarding baby care and his early involvement with the baby.
- Prepare your older child for the baby's birth and the needs of a breastfeeding baby.
- Encourage sibling involvement with the new baby and plan to spend time alone with each child.
- Learn to deal with people who are not supportive of breastfeeding.

11

Breastfeeding As Your Baby Grows

After the first few months of breastfeeding, you will probably find that your lifestyle has changed dramatically. You will, of course, have much more responsibility—but you will also share a great deal more love. Your days will be devoted to nurturing your breastfeeding relationship, adjusting to the changes in your family, and learning about your baby's special qualities. As nursing progresses, you will continue adapting breastfeeding to your lifestyle, and adjusting your activities to meet the changing needs of your maturing baby.

RESUMING SOCIAL ACTIVITIES

A major concern for many women when they consider whether or not to breastfeed is the resumption of their previous social routines. It is reassuring to know that you will be able to continue your social activities during the months that you are breastfeeding. On many occasions, you will be able to take your baby with you. If you wear appropriate clothing and choose the time and place carefully, you can discreetly nurse your baby in most situations. Sometimes, however, you will want to spend time away from your baby. While this may happen only occasionally, and for short periods, you will feel more comfortable about your baby's well-being if you know he will accept a substitute feeding while you are away. By preparing for these separations, both you and your baby are likely to be satisfied.

Taking Your Baby With You

If you remain flexible and willing to make adjustments in your usual schedule, you will be able to return to your normal routine quite successfully, and to include your baby in your activities. This will not only make your own life more fulfilling, but will enrich your baby's life by exposing him to a variety of surroundings and people.

Young babies are very portable, and breastfeeding makes travelling even easier by eliminating the need to transport bottles for feedings. Keep your baby's normal feeding schedule in mind, and plan to nurse him just before you leave. If you will be away from home during the next regular feeding, you can anticipate this and find a private place to nurse your baby.

Young babies are usually willing to sleep anywhere, so there should not be any interference with nap times. Be considerate of others if your baby does begin to cry and disturb those around you. Most people will accept your baby's presence as long as it doesn't interfere with the tasks that need to be accomplished.

A baby who has not yet learned to creep or crawl is easier to take with you than a toddler who might cause a disturbance. As your baby grows older and becomes more active, you will need to re-evaluate the types of activities that are appropriate for him. He may be better accepted as a toddler if he was included in your activities as an infant; others will have become accustomed to his presence, and perhaps will be willing to accommodate his new behavior.

Practicing Discreet Nursing

At times, you will need to nurse your baby in the presence of visitors or in places other than your own home. With planning, you will be able to breastfeed without drawing attention to yourself or offending others. You may want to practice discreet nursing at home in front of your mate or before a mirror. It may also be helpful to observe other women nursing their babies. Through practice and observation, you will gradually learn what works best for you.

Wearing Appropriate Clothing

The careful selection of clothing will enable you to nurse your baby without unnecessarily exposing your breasts. Two-piece outfits will allow you to pull your blouse up from the bottom so that the upper portion of your breast remains concealed while your baby nurses. When wearing a blouse that has buttons, open the bottom two or three buttons so that the blouse can be raised easily. To avoid fumbling with fasteners, select a nursing bra with flaps that can be fastened and unfastened with one hand. While you are nursing, your baby will cover your stomach area, and a sweater, jacket, shawl, or poncho can be used to conceal the underarm area. Another option is to drape a blanket over your baby while he is at the breast. Be sure to use a blanket that is large enough to cover both your shoulder and stomach.

Choosing the Right Location and Time

When you nurse your baby in a public area, try to find a quiet place that is out of the mainstream of activity. This will make it easier for you to relax, and will be less distracting for your curious baby. Many stores have lounge areas in their ladies' rest rooms. If not, you can ask to use a dressing room in the ladies' clothing department. You might also find it comfortable to nurse in your parked car. However, never nurse your baby while riding in a car. All small children should be restrained in approved car seats. If your baby cries and seems unable to wait for you to reach your destination without nursing, stop the car in a parking area and nurse; then return him to his car seat.

When you are out in public, try to anticipate your baby's needs and feed him before he becomes too hungry. This will allow you to position him at the breast before he attracts attention by crying. Be aware that babies draw people like magnets. Most people will not realize you are nursing, and may approach you to see your baby. You can smile and tell them that he is sleeping and can't be disturbed. Few people will insist on waking a sleeping baby!

Managing Occasional Separations

Once your baby is old enough to be left with others for short periods, you and your mate may wish to go out together and leave your baby at home. Or, perhaps, you will want some much-needed time alone for a special activity. As your baby grows older, there will probably be more and more short periods of separation. During these separations, breast milk or formula can be given in a cup or bottle. In addition to satisfying your baby's needs, be sure to consider your own comfort and to take proper care of your breasts during your absence.

In anticipation of separations, you can periodically pump or express your milk at home and save it for times when you will be away. (See Chapter 15 for complete instructions on pumping and storing breast milk.) If you prefer that your baby be given formula rather than breast milk while you are away, check with his doctor about the type that should be offered.

Generally, it is best to avoid the use of bottles with breastfed babies. However, some mothers wish to add bottle feedings to their routines. Care needs to be taken when bottles are begun. If you introduce a bottle too soon or use it too frequently, you may interfere with the building of your milk supply. In addition, your baby may become confused by the different sucking technique required. Because it is easier for him to extract milk from a bottle, he may begin to prefer that feeding method. If you wait too long, however, your baby may refuse a bottle. Many mothers have found that it is best to offer a bottle when the baby is between two and three months of age. At that time, the milk supply is well-established and, while the baby has already learned the correct method of suckling, he is still young enough to adjust to bottle feedings. Experiment with different types and shapes of nipples until you find the one your baby will accept.

Some babies will tolerate a bottle only under certain conditions. Feedings may be more successful if you have someone else give the bottle to your baby, since he may be reluctant to accept anything from you but the "real thing"! You might want to practice with a few short trial runs when your mate or another family member can stay at home and feed your baby. For your peace of mind, as well as the health and happiness of your baby, the person you select to care for him should be supportive of your breastfeeding and understanding of your needs.

In order to best satisfy your baby and maintain your milk supply, nurse him just before you leave. If you are absent during your baby's next regular feeding time, empty your breasts manually while you are away to avoid overfullness and the possibility of developing a plugged duct. No more than four hours should pass without your expressing milk to relieve the fullness in your breasts. For more information on how to manage separations, see Chapter 13 for a detailed discussion of working and nursing.

CHANGING NURSING PATTERNS AS YOUR BABY MATURES

In the later months of breastfeeding, you may encounter temporary difficulties at various stages of your baby's development. Teething and an increased awareness of his surroundings may distract your baby while he is nursing, resulting in nursing problems. These, and other changes in the breastfeeding relationship that occur as your baby grows, can be dealt with effectively when you have a clear understanding of what to expect.

Handling Teething and Biting

The eruption of teeth through gum tissue causes babies varying degrees of discomfort. Although some babies barely seem to notice the process, others suffer with each new tooth. While teething can affect breastfeeding in a variety of ways, you will be able to eliminate most problems by relieving your baby's discomfort.

It is natural for babies to chew and even bite during infancy. This is usually not a cause for concern. However, if your baby chews and bites during feedings, your nipples may become irritated. While teething is one cause of biting, many times babies bite as a result of developmental changes. A few simple precautions will keep this behavior from interfering with breastfeeding.

Soothing Your Baby During Teething

You can soothe your baby's sore gums and make it more comfortable for him to nurse by rubbing his gums with your finger or a cool cloth. You can also hold an ice cube against his gums, rub them with a spoon, or allow him to chew on a spoon or teething ring that has been cooled in the refrigerator. Although over-the-counter products for teething pain may be helpful, they cause upset stomachs in some babies. Consult your doctor before purchasing any medicated products. Once treatment has relieved your baby's discomfort, he should be able to nurse with less difficulty.

Relieving Breast Discomforts During Teething

When your baby teethes, you may find that your nipples become sore because of the enzymes present in his saliva. Cleansing your nipples with plain water after nursings will help you to avoid this irritation. Suckling may produce pain and tingling in your baby's gums, causing him to suddenly pull away from your breast. To avoid nipple stress and irritation, be ready to break suction before this happens. If your baby develops a habit of clamping down on your nipple at the end of a feeding, anticipate his actions and insert your finger between his gums to break suction before he can damage the nipple tissues. Because of the pain in his gums, your baby may cut feedings short. Since this can cause overfullness in your breasts, pump or hand express your milk whenever your baby ends a feeding prematurely.

Dealing With Biting

Biting during nursings may begin even in the absence of teething, and should be dealt with immediately. Calmly stop the feeding with a firm "No!" Your baby will soon learn that you will not allow him to continue nursing if he bites. Try to anticipate his biting, and be prepared to remove your baby from the breast as soon as he ends a feeding. Babies cannot nurse and bite at the same time; if your baby bites your nipple, it may indicate that he is no longer interested in suckling.

It is normal to jerk away and cry out the first time biting happens. Your sudden reaction by itself may be unpleasant enough to keep your baby from biting again. However, if you overreact, you may frighten your baby and cause him to fear nursing. Try to regain your composure as quickly as possible and soothe him.

Some babies close their jaws when they fall asleep at the breast. This habit can cause nipple pain and soreness, and should be discouraged. If your baby's biting at the end of a feeding becomes a problem, remove the nipple from his mouth as soon as he becomes drowsy. Also avoid snack nursings; because many babies view this as a playful time, they may bite rather than nurse.

When Your Baby Seems to Lose Interest in Nursing

Sometimes, a breast-fed baby appears to lose interest in breastfeeding. He may be easily distracted and abruptly end feedings, or may refuse to nurse at all. When this happens, you will probably become very frustrated, wondering if he is not getting enough to eat, if he wants to wean, or if he is ill. Such loss of interest in breastfeeding is usually temporary. Many babies will return to the breast after some changes have been made in the nursing routine.

Encouraging a Distracted Baby

When your baby reaches four to six months of age, you will probably observe many changes in your nursing relationship. Your body will have fully recovered from childbirth, and you and your baby will have become a well-tuned breastfeeding couple. Your child will be totally adorable and, at about this time, he may begin to experience an exciting spurt in his mental development. Isn't this what every mother waits for? It is this developmental leap, however, that will make your baby easily distracted when breastfeeding. Teething and the introduction of solid foods may also contribute to a lessening of interest in nursing at this time.

If your baby becomes distracted, make every effort to reduce interruptions and diversions by nursing in a dark, quiet room, away from family activities. You may be able to arrange only one or two uninterrupted feedings a day during this time in your baby's development. While it may be frustrating, you should view this new nursing pattern as a sign of your child's mental growth, and learn to accept the changes in your relationship.

Getting Through Nursing Strikes

At around seven months of age, some babies suddenly stop breastfeeding. This **strike**, or failure to nurse, is often related to a specific cause, such as teething; an ear infection, cold, or other illness; a leap in mental or physical development; or a reduced milk supply. Sometimes, however, you may be unable to determine the reason for the strike. Fortunately, most babies return to breastfeeding; occasionally, a baby permanently weans as a result of a nursing strike.

A sudden refusal to nurse can be very upsetting to both mother and baby. If this happens to you, you will need to find an alternative way of feeding your baby while trying to determine the reason for the nursing strike. Check for any physical problems that may have caused your baby to refuse to nurse, and have the condition treated. Your baby will probably return to breastfeeding when the symptoms disappear. During strikes, you will need to make an extra effort to maintain your milk supply. Be sure to pump or hand express milk when feedings are missed or cut short. Get plenty of rest, and eat a balanced diet with sufficient liquids.

You may have to devote several days to renewing your baby's interest in breastfeeding, and it may take as long as two weeks to return to total breastfeeding. Let your family and friends know about your plans, and ask for their support and assistance. There are a number of techniques that may help you to coax your baby back to the breast.

- Massage your breasts before attempting to nurse so that the milk will let down quickly.
- Express breast milk directly into your baby's mouth.
- Insert your nipple into your baby's mouth when he is drowsy or sleeping.
- Offer the baby your breast frequently.
- Increase evening and nighttime nursings.
- Nurse in a dark room with no distractions.
- Increase skin-to-skin contact with your baby.
- Limit or eliminate solids and other supplements.
- Offer liquids by cup, spoon, or eyedropper, rather than giving your baby a bottle.
- Avoid the use of pacifiers.
- Arrange for your baby to see other babies nursing.

If your efforts to resume breastfeeding fail, accept this as a step forward in your baby's development. Your nursing relationship will have provided him with warmth, security, and nourishment, and he will now be ready to move on to new challenges and experiences.

Nursing Your Older Baby

While breastfeeding is generally accepted as natural and appropriate, mothers who continue to nurse when their babies are beyond a socially acceptable age are often regarded with disapproval. This is unfortunate, since babies can benefit from breast milk and the breastfeeding relationship long after their first year. Your baby will continue to receive valuable nutrition from your breast milk, and the lasting closeness between you and your child will help to balance his desire for independence. In addition, breastfeeding will continue to satisfy his sucking needs, which may persist through the second year.

As your baby grows, nursings will become less frequent, and their time and location can be chosen on the basis of convenience and privacy. If your toddler is old enough, you can reason with him about appropriate ways to request to nurse. Adopt a special word for "nurse" that is not obvious to others. Arrange your nursings in a way that makes them less noticeable, or limit nursings to a secluded area of your home.

With common sense and discretion, you will be able to prevent conflicts with friends and family even as you continue the breastfeeding relationship. Avoid situations in which your nursing might be criticized by others, and refrain from discussing breastfeeding with people who object to it. If asked when you are planning to wean, explain that you have begun the gradual weaning process. If your mate objects to your nursing when your baby is older, talk to him about his specific objections and seek a compromise. Plan feedings so that you do not nurse in front of him, and refrain from complaining to him about any minor problems you may be having with breastfeeding. Discuss your baby's growth and development. Your mate may be more accepting of an extended nursing period when he understands that a baby's needs for sucking and reassurance continue as he moves toward independence.

AT A GLANCE

Breastfeeding As Your Baby Grows

Adapting Breastfeeding to Your Lifestyle

- Babies can be taken on many social outings.
- With appropriate clothing and a careful choice of location, it is possible to nurse discreetly in public.
- Breast milk or formula can be left for your baby to allow occasional separations.
- When feedings are missed, empty your breasts to avoid overfullness.
- An older baby can still derive benefits from breastfeeding. Avoid people who are unsupportive, and arrange nursings so that they are unlikely to provoke criticism.

Overcoming Roadblocks

- Teething can cause your baby discomfort when he nurses.
- To relieve teething discomfort, massage your baby's gums, give him a cooled teething ring, or try medications recommended by your doctor.
- Babies cannot bite and nurse at the same time; remove your baby from the breast when he begins biting.
- If your baby becomes distracted at the breast, nurse in a dark, quiet room.
- Babies sometimes refuse to nurse for a period of time; most return to breastfeeding when measures are taken to coax them back to the breast.

12 Your Baby's Nutritional Milestones

As your baby grows and gains weight, his nutritional needs will increase and—in time—he will require more than breast milk. Because babies vary in their need for solid foods, this milestone may be reached when your child is only four months of age, or may not appear until he is several months older.

By expanding your baby's diet to include sources of nourishment other than breast milk, the first feeding of solids will signal the earliest stage of weaning. When undertaken gradually and lovingly, the introduction of solid foods and the weaning process will blend together to move your child forward in his physical and emotional development.

INTRODUCING SOLID FOODS

A variety of factors will influence the introduction of solid foods into your baby's diet. Most parents' primary question is the proper age at which this type of feeding should begin. You may also be concerned about the best way to begin these feedings and the best kinds of foods that should initially be introduced. With patience and flexibility, you and your baby will develop a method that fits your individual needs.

Knowing When to Start Solids

The American Academy of Pediatrics recommends that solid foods be delayed until your baby is four to six months of age, whether he is breastfed or formula-fed.[1] This new recommendation may be a source of confusion, because your family, friends, and perhaps even your own physician may suggest that you begin solids earlier. The academy's guidelines were developed because of a growing concern over the development of allergies and obesity in infants and young children. There is a chance that your baby's system will be unable to handle some new foods at a very young age. Evidence points to the fact that delaying the introduction of solids until four to six months will help you to avoid or delay food allergies in your baby, or at least will reduce their seriousness.

Introducing solid foods too early may also interfere with breastfeeding success. As soon as you begin substituting solid foods for breast milk, your baby will require fewer nursings. Eventually, this will result in a lower milk supply. By introducing solid foods at a later age, after your milk supply has been well-established, you will avoid the possibility of undermining breastfeeding. If your four-month-old is still hungry after feedings, and continues to be fussy and unsatisfied despite increased nursings, he may be ready to begin eating solid foods.

Developmental milestones are even more important indicators of an infant's readiness for new foods. Your baby will gradually show signs of his capacity to eat and sit independently, including improved eye-hand coordination and the ability to grasp objects with his thumb and forefinger. By four to five months of age, the reflex that causes him to automatically push food out of his mouth will have disappeared, and he should be able to swallow food easily. By five to six months of age, he may show a desire for food by leaning forward and opening his mouth. If he does not want the food, he will be able to lean backward or turn away. In addition, a more mature intestinal system will help your child handle new types of nourishment, and his own immune system will be capable of producing the antibodies he previously received from breast milk. The most obvious sign of readiness, however, will be an interest in table foods. When you and others in your family are eating, your baby will let you know that he wants to be included.

Making a Gradual Transition to Solids

The process of introducing solid foods should be a gradual one. Initially, breast milk will continue to be your baby's main source of nourishment. Since his interest in solids may vary from day to day, you can feel confident that he is receiving all necessary nutrients from your milk. Nursing will also give your baby a sense of security as he tries new foods. To avoid the risk of decreasing your milk supply during this learning period, always nurse your baby before feeding him solids.

When your child is around six months of age, begin slowly, offering a small amount of highly pureed and diluted food at one feeding every other day. Try to view this experience as a fun, learning time for the two of you. One or two tablespoons of food are all you will have to prepare at first. If most of the food ends up *on* your baby instead of *in* him, or if he refuses to cooperate, acccept this as part of the learning process and keep trying. Feed your baby one single-ingredient food for an entire week before beginning another food. This will make it easier for you to determine if he is allergic to each new food. As your baby matures, increase the size of the food particles and dilute the food with less liquid.

When your child is seven to nine months old, he may have one or two solid feedings a day. By nine to twelve months of age, he probably will be eating three regular meals, plus snacks. While you and he may also want to continue nursing during the day, nursings can gradually be eliminated as your baby's meals become well-balanced and he begins drinking from a cup.

If you wait until four to six months to introduce solids, there is probably no specific food that should be offered first. Foods that are high in protein are a good choice for the breast-fed baby, as breast milk is lower in protein than formula. If your doctor suggests a single grain cereal, you can easily mix small amounts of it with breast milk or water. If using prepared baby foods, pour a small portion into a feeding dish and discard anything that's left in the bowl. Do not feed directly from the jar, as this will contaminate the food that remains in the jar by bringing it in contact with the saliva that clings to the spoon.

When your baby reaches about eight months of age, he will be able to grasp his food and to chew and swallow it with greater ease. At this point, you can give him soft, easy-to-swallow foods—cooked carrots, green beans, bread, etc.—that he can feed himself. This will be an exciting time for your baby, and his ability to explore the foods he is eating will help him develop many areas of awareness that are important to his mental and physical growth.

Commercial Versus Homemade Foods

You may wonder whether you should buy prepared baby foods or make your own. There are advantages and disadvantages to each option. Your own lifestyle and personal preference will determine which suits you and your baby best.

Commercially prepared baby foods are convenient, and the levels of salt and sugar have been reduced over the past few years so that they present less cause for concern than they once did. These products are easy to store and come in a wide variety to satisfy the tastes of most babies. They are expensive, however, and in the early days of introducing solids, you may find that you have to throw away quite a bit of food. Be aware that single-ingredient infant foods contain fewer additives than junior foods, which are more likely to have fillers and thickeners of questionable value.

When homemade baby foods are prepared from fresh or frozen foods, they contain few or no additives. You can prepare them in the amount your baby needs and then, using a baby food grinder, blender, or food processor, puree the foods directly from your table. You can also prepare large amounts of food and freeze them in ice cube trays or drop portions onto cookie sheets, storing the portions in a plastic bag after freezing. When prepared in large quantities from table food, homemade baby food can be considerably less expensive than commercial food. If you find it too time consuming or inconvenient to prepare all your baby's foods, a combination of the two types—commercial and homemade—may be the answer.

Your Baby's Reactions to Solid Foods

Because new foods sometimes cause babies to develop allergies, it is important for you to recognize the symptoms of an allergic reaction. Common signs of allergies include:

- Skin rashes.
- A runny, stuffy nose.
- Red, itchy eyes.
- Dark circles under the eyes.
- An upset stomach.
- General fussiness.

Since these reactions could also indicate other physical problems, you should consult your baby's doctor if these symptoms continue after you have stopped feeding your child a new food. Allergies are caused by a specific level of exposure to a substance. This level may be reached after many small exposures; therefore your child may develop an allergy to a food you have been giving him for some time without his having shown any earlier symptoms. More serious allergic reactions include asthma, recurrent ear infections, and poor weight gain. If your baby develops any of these symptoms, take him to his doctor for immediate treatment.

If either your family or your mate's family has a history of allergies, you should be particularly careful. Be sure to monitor your own diet as well as the foods your baby eats. Since many food components are present in your milk, allergens that pass through your milk may establish a sensitivity to these foods in your baby, causing an allergic reaction when they are later introduced directly to him. A history of allergies also makes it more important for you to start only one single-ingredient food at a time, and to wait at least one week before introducing another food. Cow's milk is the most common allergen; citrus fruits, eggs, wheat, fish, pork, and nuts may also cause allergic rections. See page 43, for a more detailed discussion of the breastfeeding mother's diet.

When your baby is about ten months old, he may begin to refuse new foods. By letting him take an active part in his own feedings, you may be able to overcome this behavior. At this age, your child's need to explore his world will be strong. Take advantage of his curiosity and growing abilities by giving him foods that he can handle on his own. Although these initial self-feedings will probably be long and messy, the eventual results will be worth the fuss. Continue nursing during this stage to make sure that his nutritional, sucking, and emotional needs are being met.

WEANING YOUR BABY

Once solid foods have become an established part of your baby's diet, you may wonder if it is time for weaning. Babies under one year of age still benefit from the closeness of breastfeeding, which provides a feeling of stability and security. They also continue to have a strong need for sucking and, in some cases, a fear of being separated from their mothers. Weaning should be considered only after these needs have been met, motor skills have been mastered, and a regular meal pattern has been established.

Although a situation may arise that calls for immediate weaning, a slow weaning process is best for your baby. Ideally, he will gradually wean himself as he begins to rely more on solid foods for his nourishment and becomes more involved in activities other than breastfeeding. However, you may feel that you are ready to end breastfeeding before your baby shows signs of weaning. Both your needs and his should be considered. Pressure from others should not influence your decision or cause you to wean when you do not feel that the time is right.

Regardless of the circumstances surrounding the weaning

process, you and your baby will have emotional and physical adjustments to make, and both of you will probably have mixed reactions to this change in your relationship. Accept your feelings and his. In time, you will find that the weaning process is a period of growth during which your relationship broadens to encompass new experiences and activities.

Baby-Led Weaning

Weaning will be most successful if your baby is allowed to decide when it will take place. You may have hoped to continue nursing for a longer period of time. If your baby is under nine months of age, the discussion of nursing strikes on page 166 may help you to coax your baby back to breastfeeding. However, signs of weaning in an older baby should be accepted as an indication of his readiness to take a new step in his development. If he is ready to wean, his needs should be considered before your own. Do not insist on his breastfeeding when he is not interested.

Your baby's readiness for weaning will reflect his increased ability to cope with the world outside the breastfeeding relationship. Solid foods will have become well-established in his feeding pattern, and he may be easily distracted when nursing. When he asks to nurse, he may very quickly change his mind, because his main interest is in the world around him.

Baby-led weaning is the most desirable method because it allows your baby to satisfy his needs at his own pace. Although an increase in the frequency of nursings may occasionally occur, you will detect a gradual lessening of your child's desire to breastfeed. Ideally, the nursing relationship will end slowly and lovingly over a period of time.

Mother-Led Weaning

Your own needs in the nursing relationship are also an important consideration. If nursing an older baby makes you feel anxious or resentful, you may wish to begin the weaning process without cues from your child.

If weaning begins when your baby is under one year of age, you should substitute bottle feeding for breastfeeding to ensure that his sucking needs will still be met. Mother-led weaning should take place over several weeks. At times, your baby may readily accept alternatives to breastfeeding. At other times, when he is upset or ill, he may refuse everything but the breast. Respond to these occasional setbacks with plenty of love and patience, for they are a natural part of the weaning process. If you choose to initiate weaning, the following suggestions may help both you and your baby to feel more comfortable during the transitional period.

- Eliminate the least preferred nursing first.
- Slowly drop other nursings—one at a time, over several days—eliminating your baby's favorite feeding last.
- Provide other types of food and drink when your baby asks to nurse.
- Involve your baby in activities that he enjoys, and find acceptable substitutes for nursing (e.g., playing games, reading books, and assembling puzzles).
- Provide your baby with attention and closeness in other ways and at other times. By cuddling him, singing to him, and taking walks with him, you can give your child the affection that he needs.
- Stretch the time between nursings, telling your toddler, "We will nurse in a few minutes" or "We'll nurse after we finish our chores."
- Avoid using nursing to soothe every hurt or distressing situation.
- Be aware of any uncomfortable fullness in your breasts, and pump or express only enough to relieve discomfort. Too much pumping will encourage milk production.

Emergency Weaning

If an emergency requires that you wean quickly, be careful to avoid overfullness, which could lead to a plugged duct or breast infection. Binding your breasts is not recommended, since it may result in plugged ducts and can be terribly painful. The effects of lactation suppressants are often only temporary, and lactation may resume after a few days. If emergency weaning is necessary, the following suggestions may help to ease the transition from breastfeeding to bottle or cup feeding.

- When possible, take at least two days to complete the weaning process. On the first day, eliminate every other nursing. On the second day, eliminate all nursings.
- Substitute a bottle or cup—whichever is more acceptable.
- Express to relieve fullness. To avoid further milk production, express no more than one or two ounces at a time.
- Use ice packs to relieve the pain of engorgement.

Adjustments to Weaning

The weaning process will require a number of adjustments on the part of both you and your baby. Occasionally, you may find that your baby wants to return to more frequent nursings. Such a regression should be handled lovingly and with the knowledge that your child will soon return to his former pattern.

You, too, may experience mixed feelings about the change in your relationship with your baby. You may enioy the freedom from the responsibility of nursing, but at the same time regret the loss of intimacy. Before long, you and your baby will discover new interests to share.

Regressions During Weaning

Occasionally, an older baby will seem to be nearly weaned and then suddenly increase his nursings. You may be discouraged by this step backward and wonder what went wrong. Sometimes, regression will occur when your baby is ill, or when new events or accomplishments cause him to feel a need for reassurance. Or it may be that weaning was taking place too fast for him, and was not allowing for a comfortable period of adjustment.

Let him nurse at his own pace for a day or two, and then resume the weaning process more slowly. Be sure to provide him with extra attention during this stressful time. A return to frequent nursings is usually temporary. If you provide other forms of stimulation and attention, recognizing your baby's immediate needs, he will again begin to accept a decrease in nursings. Acknowledge your child's ability to amuse himself, and encourage his involvement in activities other than nursing.

Your Physical and Emotional Reactions to Weaning

A variety of physical and emotional changes may accompany the weaning process. You may feel a sense of loss because of the change in your relationship with your child. As he becomes more independent, he may appear to need you less. It is normal to have some regrets about this new stage in your child's development. You will find, however, that both of you will move forward to new experiences, and that his dependence on you will manifest itself in new ways.

Once your baby is completely weaned, you will begin to notice changes in your body. It may take several months before you stop producing breast milk, depending on hormonal levels and the amount of stimulation your nipples receive. Your breasts will soon begin to return to their prepregnant size, appearing droopy at first, but eventually regaining their firmness. In addition, the Montgomery glands will recede. If you have not already resumed your normal menstrual cycle, you should begin regular menstruation shortly after weaning.

When weaning begins, you can avoid weight gain by reducing your calorie intake. Your baby will no longer be helping you to utilize the extra calories included in your diet during pregnancy and lactation. Omit the extra foods and reduce portion sizes, but do not forget the sound nutritional practices that were part of your pregnancy and breastfeeding regimen. Continue to select foods wisely and to make good nutrition a priority for you and your family.

AT A GLANCE

Your Baby's Nutritional Milestones

Introducing Solid Foods Into Your Baby's Diet

- The introduction of solid foods should be delayed until 4 to 6 months age.
- By 6 months, most babies begin to show signs that they are ready to begin eating solids.
- Solid foods should be introduced gradually, in small amounts of single-ingredient foods.
- If your family has a history of food allergies, carefully monitor the foods you eat, as well as those you give to your baby.
- Allergic reactions to foods are characterized by skin rashes; a runny, stuffy nose; red, itchy eyes; circles under the eyes; an upset stomach; and fussiness. If your baby shows any of these symptoms, the solid food that has been most recently introduced should be eliminated from his diet.
- Homemade baby foods are inexpensive, contain few or no additives, and are easy to prepare with a baby food grinder or blender.
- Commercially prepared baby foods are convenient, but more expensive. Low salt and sugar levels make them an acceptable option. Choose single-ingredient foods that do not contain fillers and additives.
- Always nurse before giving your baby solid foods.
- By 9 to 12 months, your baby may be eating three regular meals, with snacks, daily.

When to Wean Your Baby

- Weaning should begin when you and your baby are ready, and not as result of pressure from others.
- Weaning is best accomplished when it is initiated by the baby.

- Your baby will probably be ready for weaning when solid foods are a regular part of his diet, he is easily distracted during feedings, and his nursings are infrequent.
- Mother-led weaning—weaning that you initiate without cues from your baby—can also enjoy success.

How to Wean Your Baby

- To initiate weaning, slowly reduce the number of feedings over several days, provide other forms of food and drink when your baby asks to nurse, involve your baby in other activities, and find alternative ways of providing your baby with attention.
- During the weaning process, express milk if your breasts become uncomfortably full.
- If you must wean quickly, eliminate every other nursing on the first day and the remaining nursings on the second day; express milk to relieve fullness; and apply ice packs to your breasts to relieve pain.
- Your baby may exhibit some regression during the weaning process; respond to his needs by allowing additional nursings.
- If your baby weans before he reaches one year of age, he should be weaned to a bottle to satisfy his sucking needs.
- As your baby weans, reduce your food consumption to avoid gaining weight.
- It is normal to feel some sadness when your baby weans. Accept weaning as a positive step in your child's development, and find new activities and interests to share with him.

13
Managing Working and Nursing

An increasing number of women are now working outside the home, and many of these women have young children. A mother has special needs when balancing child care and work, and these needs increase when she chooses to breastfeed. If you decide to continue breastfeeding after returning to work, you will have many options to consider and plans to make. Become as knowledgeable as possible about breastfeeding in order to determine your own personal goals and priorities. As your baby grows, his needs will change, necessitating a continual re-evaluation of your objectives throughout your breastfeeding experience.

PREPARING FOR YOUR RETURN

Once you have made the decision to return to work and to continue breastfeeding, you should set a date for your return and prepare yourself and your baby for your new routine. You will benefit from supportive home and work environments; take steps to ensure that they will contribute as little stress as possible to your life while you make the necessary adjustments. In addition, you will have to explore the available types of child care and to choose the one that is most compatible with your breastfeeding and parenting goals. By making these plans early and preparing yourself and your baby, you will increase your chance of successfully combining breastfeeding and working.

Time Your Return With Baby in Mind

Realistically, you may have no choice about when you will return to work. If your situation permits it, however, plan your return so that it interferes as little as possible with breastfeeding. Although there is no ideal age at which a baby can be separated from his mother, it is best to delay the separation until your baby is at least six to eight weeks old, a time when your milk supply is firmly established. If you return to work at this point, you will have a good chance for success. If you can delay your return even further—until your baby is four to six months old and has begun eating solid foods—the transition will be all the easier.

Build a Supportive Environment

To some degree, your success will depend on the aid and encouragement you receive from the people who are closest to you. Your partner's support is most important, as priorities at home will have to accommodate you and your baby. Let your mate know how much you will benefit from his emotional support, as well as his practical help with household chores.

At work, make your employer aware of your special needs as they relate to breastfeeding, being sure he or she knows that you will not allow breastfeeding to interfere with job performance. An unsupportive work environment can compromise your ability to nurse successfully, so try to avoid conflicts or to resolve them before they affect your nursing.

Another invaluable source of support is available to you through local breastfeeding groups. Seek out such a group in your community and establish contact with a volunteer counselor. If no such group exists in your community, perhaps you can enlist support from your childbirth instructor or another interested professional.

Evaluate Possible Work Arrangements

Some work schedules are more conducive to breastfeeding than others. Check with your employer to find out what options are available. If you plan to work outside your home, you may want to consider the following alternatives to standard full-time employment:

- Flextime, whereby you choose hours that fit into your personal schedule.
- Part-time employment, with work hours planned around your baby's nursing and sleeping schedule and other family-related responsibilities.
- Working part of the time at the job location, and the remainder of the time at home.
- Sharing a full-time position with another person, so that each of you works on a part-time basis.

If possible, choose arrangements such as flextime and part-time employment, as they will not take you away from your baby for long periods. Also consider the location of your job. If you work near the place where your baby is being cared for, you may be able to provide feedings throughout the day.

Review Child Care Options

Finding good child care takes time and effort. In light of your decision to breastfeed, you should select a person to care for your baby who will follow your directions and who is supportive of your decision to continue nursing. Alternatives you may wish to consider are:

- Your baby's father. Perhaps you can coordinate both work schedules so that one of you will always be at home with your baby.
- A sitter who comes to your home. This will allow your baby to remain comfortable in a familiar environment.
- A sitter who cares for the baby at her own home. If your sitter lives in close proximity to your job, you may be able to nurse your baby during breaks.
- A day care center. Once you are satisfied that your baby's physical needs will be met, carefully examine the interaction between the staff members, parents, and children.

Your return to work will go more smoothly if you first conduct one or more trial runs with your baby sitter. Start by leaving for short periods, and gradually increase the time you stay away. Introducing your baby to his sitter in this way will help him adjust more easily and will enable you to determine whether or not you are comfortable with the arrangement. It is a good idea to schedule these trial runs several weeks before your return to work. If the first sitter is not satisfactory, you will still have time to make other arrangements.

Once you have made your decision, familiarize your sitter with some of the special aspects of breastfeeding. If your baby will be given relief bottles of breast milk, rather than formula, describe the normal appearance of breast milk, and the more frequent feedings required by a breast-fed baby. Regardless of the type of feeding your sitter will be providing, she should learn about the nature of a breast-fed baby's stools, and the need to have your baby eager to nurse when you return.

Practice Expressing Milk

Before you return to work, practice expressing your breast milk at home so that you will be able to do it with ease once you are working. Do not become discouraged if you fail to express much milk at first. The purpose of these sessions is to refine your technique. The quantity of milk will increase with practice.

Use either manual expression or a breast pump, saving any milk you express and freezing it for later use. Try to collect and freeze a substantial supply during the weeks before your return to work; you will then have a reserve for those times when you are unable to express milk. It may take an entire day to fill a four-ounce bottle, pouring one layer onto the next until the bottle is full. To prevent the production of excessive quantities of milk during your first days at work, discontinue these home pumping sessions several days before your return.

Offer Bottles to Your Baby

In the weeks before you return to work, periodically offer your baby a bottle to ensure that he will accept one when you are away. Since he is accustomed to nursing from your breast, he may not accept a bottle from you; however, he may be more responsive if someone else feeds him. If your baby refuses the bottle initially, experiment with various types of nipples until you find one that he will accept. Be assured that most breast-fed babies will take a bottle when they are really hungry and mother is not around.

MANAGING AT WORK

Once you return to work, your breastfeeding success will greatly depend on your ability to maintain your milk supply. If you plan to provide your baby with relief bottles of breast milk, the establishment of a satisfactory feeding routine will also depend on your success in expressing and storing milk. The general guidelines presented here should be tailored to fit your own particular needs and circumstances. Flexibility and creativity will help you and your baby to adapt to your new schedule.

Maintain Your Milk Supply

In order to continue nursing successfully, your milk supply must be well-established when the separation period begins, and must remain at an adequate level. By regularly emptying your breasts, you will ensure that sufficient milk production continues. Some women are able to maintain an adequate supply of milk by nursing in the mornings and evenings during workdays, and on a regular schedule of morning, afternoon, and evening feedings during the weekend. Others need to express milk while they are at work in order to keep up their supplies.

Expressing Breast Milk While at Work

Physical and mental relaxation will greatly enhance your success at expressing milk. Discuss your needs with your employer. Decide on the best time and location for a twenty-minute break, and explore the availability of refrigeration for the expressed milk. If you are hesitant to bring up these issues with your employer, you may be able to make satisfactory arrangements with one of your co-workers. The following guidelines should be of help as you learn to express milk at work.

- Wear clothing that will allow easy access to your breasts.
- Find a private location where you will feel comfortable and need not worry about interruptions.
- Experiment to determine how often you must express milk, taking care not to allow your breasts to become overly full.
- Drink some water, juice, or milk while you are expressing your milk, both to help you relax and to assure adequate fluid intake. Massage your breasts to initiate letdown.
- Alternate sides so that you express milk from each breast two or three times during each break.
- If letdown does not occur, take a few deep breaths, think about your baby, have something to drink, and try again.
- If your baby is not receiving breast milk during your absence, express only enough to relieve discomfort.
- Refrigerate or otherwise cool your milk while at work.

Store Breast Milk Properly

Many manual breast pumps have a bottle attachment in which you can save your milk after pumping. When using hand expression, you can express directly into a sterile baby bottle or plastic nursing bag. Recent studies indicate that breast milk can be stored safely at room temperature for up to six hours.[1] To be on the safe side, however, you should place your expressed milk in a cool place as soon as possible. If you do not have access to a refrigerator, carry a small cooler with ice. Once the milk has been heated, it should not be refrigerated again. Therefore, try to store your milk in three- to four-ounce portions—the amount your baby will use at one feeding.

The expressed breast milk can be refrigerated and fed to your baby the following day, or it may be frozen for later use. Milk can be refrigerated for up to forty-eight hours, or frozen at 0°F for up to six months. If the milk is to be saved for more than one day, it should be stored tin a sterile container. See Chapter 15 for complete information on collecting, storing, and using expressed breast milk.

Prepare for Leaking

Convenient times for milk expression may not always coincide with the times when you need to relieve the fullness in your breasts. Also, milk expression will not empty your breasts as efficiently as nursing. Consequently, you may experience some leaking while at work. There are a few measures that may help you to cope with leaking.

- Wear breast pads or breast shells if leaking is heavy. Do not wear shells all day, as they will stimulate the breast to make more milk.
- Cross your-arms and exert pressure on your breasts with the heels of your hands to temporarily stop the flow of milk. (See Figure 8.2 on page 118.)
- Wear loose-fitting patterned clothing to conceal wetness.
- Keep a sweater or jacket at work to conceal wet clothing.

MANAGING YOUR DAILY ROUTINE

When at home, your major concerns will revolve around preparing the necessary relief feedings for your baby, establishing a nursing pattern, and managing your multiple roles. Your adjustment will involve not only breastfeeding, but also the need for new priorities at home as a result of your employment. You may have to try a variety of routines before you discover the one that suits you best. You may also find that specific techniques and arrangements will work for a time, but must be changed as your baby grows and develops.

Daytime Feedings

Communicating closely with your sitter will help you to keep track of the amount of milk your baby takes during your absence. You can then determine how much milk to pump while at work and whether there is a need for formula supplements. If you are considering having your baby receive formula at the sitter's, be aware of the advantages of providing breast milk until your baby is at least three months of age. Total breastfeeding provides many allergy-preventive and disease protective elements, as well as nutritional benefits. Later, when you begin introducing solid foods and other supplements into your baby's diet you can ask the sitter to feed him these foods. This will provide more nursing time for you and your baby.

Nursing at Home

When you and your baby are together, nurse frequently to maintain your milk supply. The skin-to-skin contact will be comforting to your baby, and his contentment will help you enjoy success in your combined role of worker and breastfeeding mother. Try to nurse immediately before leaving for work, even if only a short time has passed since the previous feeding. If your baby is full when you leave, he will need less nourishment while you are at work.

To ensure that your baby will be eager to nurse when you get home, ask your sitter to avoid feeding him within one or two hours of your return. Try to nurse as soon as you and your baby are reunited and as often as your baby wishes. Frequent feedings will help to satisfy your baby's sucking needs and maintain a good milk supply.

On those days when you don't work, you may allow your baby to nurse on demand, or you may choose to maintain your workday schedule. You may even encourage night feedings so that you can spend a quiet, leisurely time with your baby without the distractions of telephones, doorbells, and other family members. These extra nursings will also help you to maintain your milk supply.

The amount of milk you produce may fluctuate between workdays and non-workdays. Even on those days when you are with your baby, your milk supply may diminish to the point where supplements are needed. This will depend on your baby's age, the length of time you have been working, and the amount of supplements that are regularly being given. You can always increase your milk supply with frequent nursings and frequent expression.

Priorities and Adjustments at Home

Your baby's welfare will undoubtedly be your number one priority. By spending your first hour home with your baby—alone, and without distractions—you will help to calm and comfort both yourself and your child. Accept offers of assistance from friends and relatives, suggesting specific tasks that they can perform to allow you to spend more time with your baby. Arrange for other family members, as well, to have special moments alone with you each day. Simplify your life by planning quiet activities at home and employing housekeeping short cuts that allow you more free time. Often, you will be able to plan social activities that include your baby so that your time together is not compromised.

It will be normal to experience some periods of frustration during your first days back at work. Flexibility, perseverance, and a sense of humor will be your greatest allies. Any change requires a period of adjustment; allow yourself time to become comfortable with your dual role as mother and working woman. The emotional benefits of breastfeeding will help you through this challenging time.

After you begin to work, you may notice changes in your baby's behavior. He may appear to reject you when you return home, or he may cling to you and demand a great deal of time and attention. Allow your baby the same adjustment period you allow yourself. Keep in mind, too, that many types of behavior are caused by developmental changes. Your baby's reactions will not necessarily be related to either your work situation or nursing.

You may, however, experience some problems that are unique to breastfeeding. Occasionally, a breast-fed baby who receives bottles regularly refuses to nurse, having developed a preference for the bottle. While this may be temporary, it could lead to permanent weaning. If this happens when your baby is young, you will probably be able to renew his interest in breastfeeding. (See page 167 for tips on coaxing your baby back to the breast.) Remember, also, that fatigue and irregular nursing patterns can lead to plugged ducts and breast infections. Take care not to allow yourself to become overly tired and to avoid any abrupt change in your nursing schedule.

At times, you may question whether you can continue to balance working and breastfeeding. Successful breastfeeding will require that you be flexible in your approach and determined to make the arrangement work. Keep a positive outlook when faced with obstacles, and maintain contact with a breastfeeding adviser. With a supportive environment, you will be able to experience the joys of breastfeeding for many months after your return to work.

AT A GLANCE

Managing Working and Nursing

Planning for Your Return to Work

- Time your return so that it is least likely to disrupt your breastfeeding relationship.
- Create a supportive environment by letting your employer, family, and friends know of your special needs.
- Re-evaluate your work arrangement, considering alternatives that might fit better into your new lifestyle.
- Review child care options, choosing a sitter or day-care center that will be supportive of your special needs.
- Begin expressing your milk, both to become comfortable with the procedure and to begin saving milk for your baby.
- Offer bottles to your baby periodically to be sure that he will accept bottle feedings.

Managing Breastfeeding at Work

- You may need to express milk regularly to maintain your milk supply.
- Facilitate milk expression by wearing appropriate clothing, selecting the right location, and using relaxation techniques.
- Express milk from both breasts, alternating sides until the flow subsides.
- Place feeding-sized portions of milk in sterile, individual bottles, and cool the milk immediately.
- Leaking may occur, but can be controlled or concealed.

Managing Your Daily Routine

- Keep track of how much your baby drinks each day so you will know how much milk to provide for his relief bottles.
- When you and your baby are together, nurse frequently to maintain your milk supply and to provide skin-to-skin contact.

- Nurse right before leaving for work and as soon as you return home. Use your first after-work nursing to renew contact with your baby.
- Your milk supply may fluctuate between workdays and non-workdays.
- Accept offers of help from friends and relatives so that you can spend more time with your baby.
- Both you and your baby will have to adjust to your work routine. Allow adequate time for this adjustment.

14
Nursing in Special Situations

While a variety of situations can make breastfeeding more difficult, many women have nursed successfully even when faced with complex problems. Circumstances that may cause a change in the normal course of breastfeeding include Cesarean birth, multiple birth, the birth of a premature or ill baby, and the hospitalization of mother or baby. If you encounter one of these situations, you may have to modify your image of the ideal breastfeeding experience or, in some cases, postpone breastfeeding. With confidence and patience, however, you should be able to overcome temporary setbacks and to establish a successful nursing relationship.

BREASTFEEDING AFTER A CESAREAN BIRTH

More babies are born by Cesarean today than ever before. In some hospitals, as many as 30 percent of the births are Cesarean. This increase in the number of mothers who have Cesareans, coupled with the increased numbers of women who choose to breastfeed, has made it necessary to develop guidelines for post-Cesarean nursing. If you are one of the many women who will experience a Cesarean delivery, take heart in the fact that you have the same chance of breastfeeding success as those women who give birth vaginally. You may, of course, experience a slower start because of your longer recovery period and the possibility of your baby's initial drowsiness. However, this should not prevent you from successfully establishing your breastfeeding relationship.

Your Own Physical Needs

In order to breastfeed after surgery, you will need help from the hospital nursing staff. Ask for assistance in adjusting the intravenous tubing so that you can hold your baby comfortably. You may also need help in positioning the baby to avoid irritating your incision. A pillow or folded blanket placed over the area will protect it from your baby's movements. The careful placement of additional pillows will further enhance your comfort.

Relax and take your time. If discomfort interferes with your ability to relax, request a pain medication that is approved for nursing mothers, and take it fifteen to twenty minutes before breastfeeding. It is often helpful to have the bedrails up when nursing, as they will provide you with support when you move your baby from one side to the other. You may find it more comfortable to nurse sitting up than lying down; experiment with different positions until you find the one you prefer.

Your baby may be drowsy as a result of the medication you received during surgery. Consequently, he may have some initial difficulty getting on the breast, or may fall asleep while nursing. Consult page 68 for ways to rouse your sleepy baby. After a day or two, your baby will be more alert and better able to nurse. The first week of breastfeeding will require perseverance and patience. Resting with your nursing baby will speed your recovery while helping to quickly establish your milk supply.

Rooming-In With Your Baby

Rooming-in is certainly possible for a Cesarean mother and her baby. Because of your need to recover from surgery, however, you may have to work up gradually to full rooming-in. On the day of your child's birth, you may be able to manage only his feedings. On the day after delivery, you may be able to manage some baby care as well. As your recovery permits, slowly increase the time you spend with your baby. Ask the staff if you can have your newborn taken back to the nursery when you feel the need for extra rest. The more flexibility you have, the more successful the arrangement is likely to be.

Your Recovery at Home

Because Cesarean birth involves major surgery, you will understandably need more time to recover from childbirth than you would after a vaginal birth. During the first weeks after delivery, it will be most important to restrict your activities to caring for your baby. Rest as much as possible, taking frequent naps. Keep all baby supplies nearby so that you can stay in bed. If you are able to get people to help you, let them take care of the household duties while you concentrate on your baby.

Good nutrition and extra fluids will be vital to your recovery. The stress of surgery reduces the levels of vitamins and minerals in your body. Since you will be establishing breastfeeding as well as recovering from surgery, you will need to be especially careful to select nutritious, well-balanced meals. By meeting your physical requirements, you will soon find that you have returned to your prepregnant level of energy, and that breastfeeding has become an important and highly rewarding part of your life.

BREASTFEEDING MORE THAN ONE BABY

We sometimes marvel at the success of women who nurse more than one baby. Many mothers of twins—and even triplets—nurse for as long as they wish, with enough milk for all babies. Breastfeeding more than one baby does present some special challenges. You must take care to eat a well-balanced diet, allow sufficient time for nursings, and get plenty of rest. Naturally, these are no easy accomplishments when you have two or three babies to care for!

Since rest is important to milk production, you should take naps whenever you have the opportunity, and relax while nursing. Performing routine baby-care tasks will be a major área of concern. Decide which jobs are most important to you, and take care of only the essentials. Solicit help in caring for other children and doing household chores. You can then devote the majority of your time to establishing breastfeeding and obtaining the rest you need.

In order to build up your milk supply initially, most of your time in the first weeks will be spent nursing your babies. With proper nutrition and sufficient fluids, you should be able to produce enough milk. Any time you feel that your milk supply is low, short frequent feedings will help to increase it. Once your supply has been established, you may wish to have someone give your babies a bottle once a day to allow you some relief from child care. Incorporating regular supplemental bottles into your babies' feeding schedules may help you to adapt breastfeeding to your daily routine.

Breastfeeding twins or triplets can be a rewarding experience for mother and babies. Take the opportunity to get to know your babies as individuals by spending some special time alone with each one. Regardless of the number of daily nursings or the number of supplemental bottles, you and your babies will benefit from your nursing relationship. As your babies grow and require less attention, you may find yourself saying, as many mothers of more than one baby do, "They were easier than having just one!"

Special Tips for Nursing Twins

Many mothers prefer nursing their twins at the same time. In this regard, you will have an advantage over formula-feeding mothers. Since you will not be encumbered by bottles, you will be able to feed two babies at the same time, and give them both the comfort of being held. This method of nursing will not only make efficient use of your time, but may also help you to coordinate your babies' feeding and sleeping schedules. If your children are on noticeably different schedules, you may have to work toward this type of feeding gradually.

Dual feedings are especially easy in the beginning, when the babies are small. At this time, you will need extra pillows to support and position your infants. See Figure 14.1 for possible ways

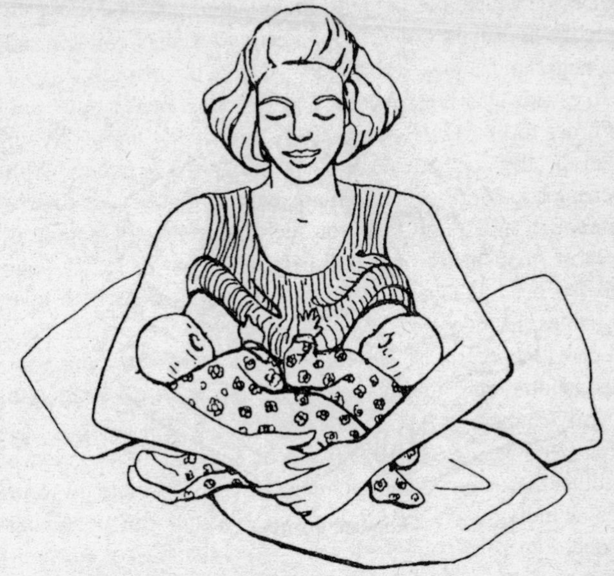

Crisscross Position

Figure 14.1 Possible Positions for Nursing Twins

to hold both babies when feeding them together. If you decide to nurse your twins together, you should still plan to feed them individually at least once a day so that each one can enjoy special time alone with you.

If you feel that nursing your twins together prevents them from receiving individual attention, you can nurse them separately. Although this method requires more time, it works well for some mothers. Your children may have growth spurts at different times and show differences in their readiness for solid foods and weaning. A combination of dual and separate feedings will enable you to respond to your babies as they grow and develop different needs.

There are a number of methods for offering the breasts at each feeding. Alternating breasts between each baby daily or at every other feeding will compensate for any differences in your babies' suckling. This will ensure equal milk production from each

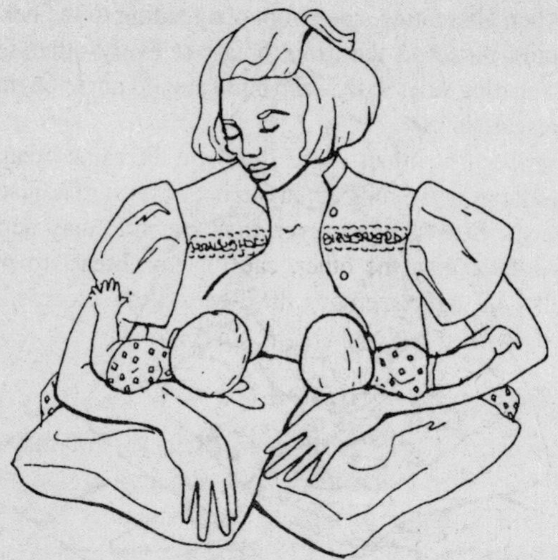

Football Position

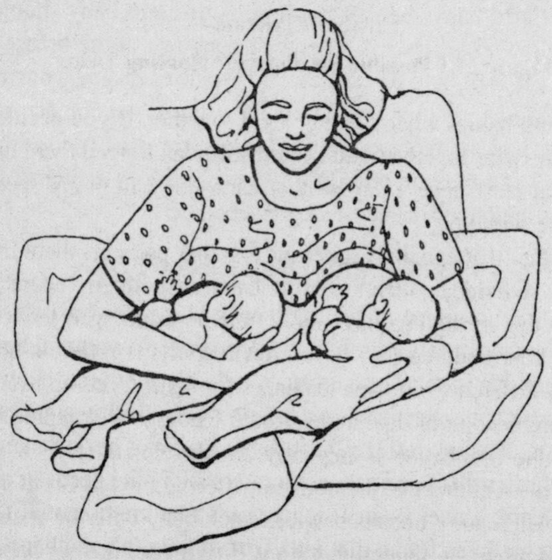

Side-by-Side Position

breast. When alternating sides from one feeding to the next, each child should nurse on the same breast at every other feeding. When alternating sides daily, each child should nurse on the same breast every other day.

A third option is to nurse each baby on the same breast at all feedings, allowing the milk supply in each breast to adjust to one baby's needs. Be aware, however, that one child may be a more vigorous nurser than the other, causing one breast to produce more milk. All three methods have been used successfully by nursing mothers.

Special Tips for Nursing Triplets

Many women have successfully nursed triplets. You may choose to totally breastfeed all babies at every feeding, or you may prefer to provide a bottle for one of your babies at each feeding while you nurse the other two. To save time and energy, a helper can give one child a bottle while you nurse the other two. After you become more experienced, you may not even need a helper for your third baby. At each feeding, a different baby should be fed with the bottle, so that all enjoy equal time at the breast.

Rest, eat well, and drink plenty of fluids to ensure your well-being and to maintain a sufficient supply of breast milk. Regardless of the feeding method, caring for triplets requires an extra pair of hands. In addition, you will have to establish clear priorities and an efficient childcare schedule.

NURSING A PREMATURE OR ILL NEWBORN

When a circumstance arises that keeps you from breastfeeding your baby directly after birth, you may wonder if you will be able to nurse at all. In most situations, it is likely that your baby will be able to nurse eventually, depending on his birth weight, overall health, sucking reflex, and the medications he is receiving. While breast milk alone may not totally satisfy the needs of a premature baby, it does contain ingredients that are essential to his health. It has been found that milk from a premie's mother is better suited to him than the milk produced by the mother of a full-term baby.[1] If your baby is premature or has some problem that makes it necessary for him to remain in the hospital for some time after birth, you can take steps to make breastfeeding possible.

Establishing a Milk Supply

To generate an adequate milk supply, begin pumping your breasts as soon as possible after delivery. Most hospitals will be able to provide you with an electric breast pump for this purpose. If you cannot obtain an electric pump, there are a variety of hand pumps on the market. See Chapter 15 for a complete discussion of breast pumps.

While in the hospital, set up a pumping schedule that is similar to the feeding schedule of a breastfeeding baby. Pump for about twenty minutes every two or three hours during the day. To further build your milk supply, continue this routine when you are home. It will not be necessary to pump at night until a week before your baby is able to nurse. If you must pump for more than two weeks, it would be best to rent an electric pump from a hospital supply store, a pharmacy, or an independent pump rental station. Ask the hospital staff if they can refer you to a local source.

Arrange for hospital personnel to provide your baby with your breast milk. Ask how much they will need, how often you should bring it, and whether it should be fresh or frozen. If you spend a good deal of time at the hospital, request that an electric pump be made available for your use while you are there. If the hospital is located far from your home, you may need a hand pump for use at some point in your trips to and from the hospital.

When you first begin pumping, you may only get a few drops of milk at each sitting. Do not be discouraged; this is perfectly normal. A premature baby requires extremely small feedings at first, so any milk you are able to collect should be sufficient. Concentrate on conditioning your letdown reflex, and continue pumping. Stimulating letdown may be easier if you tape a picture of your baby to the pump, or if you pump right after you visit him. Your persistence will be rewarded as the constant stimulation of your breasts increases your milk production.

Visiting Your Baby

Your first sight of the tubes, monitors, and other medical devices your baby needs may make you feel helpless and frightened. However, frequent visits will help both you and your newborn, especially if you can touch, fondle, and talk to him early and often. If possible, spend time alone with your baby so that the two of you can begin to develop a bond. If your baby's condition allows it, ask that you be permitted to personally provide as much of his care as you can. Be sure to get answers to any questions you have so that you will fully understand your baby's condition.

Feedings in the Hospital

You probably will be permitted to begin feedings as soon as your baby has grown stronger and can be removed from the isolette. At first, these feedings may be by bottle, but you should gradually introduce breastfeeding to your baby before you take him home. Try to be realistic about these first nursing sessions. Your baby will tire easily and won't be accustomed to this new method of obtaining nourishment. You will both need time to adjust.

When preparing to nurse, relaxation techniques will help you to achieve letdown. Because your baby will probably be small, you may need extra pillows to aid you in positioning him properly at the breast. Holding him in either the football or transverse position will give you control over his movements. You can help him to grasp the breast by gently guiding his head toward your breast with your cradling arm. Use your free hand to open his mouth by gently pushing down on his chin. Draw him close to you, and insert your nipple in his mouth. You may then wish to use the C-hold to ensure that your baby's mouth is positioned well back on the areola. If you have problems, stop and begin again. To encourage swallowing, use downward strokes under your baby's chin and talk in a soothing, coaxing tone. If your baby is not interested in the breast, try to entice him with a little expressed breast milk and plenty of skin-to-skin contact. Some mothers have been successful in using a special device to help their babies adapt to breastfeeding. See page 223 for information about the nursing supplementer.

Once your baby begins breastfeeding, he may alternately nurse and rest several times during each feeding. Allow for this, and prepare for long, relaxed times at the breast. In the beginning, you will very likely need to supplement these nursings with formula. Always offer supplements after your baby has nursed. Whatever the outcome of these in-hospital nursings, be assured that, once out of the hospital, you will enjoy greater success. The privacy and familiar surroundings afforded by your home will help you to relax and establish letdown, while the freedom from hospital procedure will give you more time to discover the positions that work best for you and your baby.

Feedings at Home

Try to prepare for your baby's discharge at least a week in advance. Pump frequently, beginning one or two pumpings during the night to build your milk supply. You will need to devise a feeding plan with your doctor, deciding on the type, amount, and frequency of formula supplements. Remember to always nurse your baby first if you are supplementing separately. Because your baby will tire easily, continue to allow long sessions at the breast so that he may rest several times during each feeding. He will nurse awhile, then rest or actually fall asleep, and then wake to nurse again. This intermittent pattern will naturally result in the short, frequent feedings that are needed to increase your milk supply.

Initially, your baby will probably be weak, and will sleep a great deal. For this reason, he may—if allowed to follow his own schedule—wait too long between feedings to receive adequate nourishment. Try to wake him every one and a half to two hours to initiate nursings. Even if he is drowsy and seems uninterested, the nipple stimulation provided by these feedings will help to increase your milk supply. More than likely, your baby will fall asleep after one breast and wake in an hour or two on his own to nurse at the second breast. During his first week at home, anticipate that most of your time will be devoted to establishing breastfeeding.

After having been bottle-fed, your baby may have trouble getting used to the breast. He can be weaned gradually from the bottle to the breast by using the following techniques.

- Before each feeding, massage your breasts and express or pump your milk until letdown occurs.
- Nurse often—every one and a half to two hours.
- Nurse more often, rather than increasing the amount of formula supplement.
- Use a nursing supplementer (see page 223) to supplement during a feeding.
- If supplementing with a bottle, offer the breast first and limit the amount of formula offered afterward.
- If a bottle is used for supplements, use an orthodontic nipple on the bottle to minimize confusion for your baby.

After a long delay in breastfeeding, you may find that you are unable to coax your baby to nurse. If you decide to continue using formula feedings alone, there is no need to feel guilty or to think you have failed. Providing your baby with breast milk in the early days was beneficial to his health. You should feel proud of your contribution.

MANAGING BREASTFEEDING DURING ILLNESS

Many nursing mothers are faced with illness at some time during their breastfeeding experiences. Fortunately, these illnesses are most often of a minor nature, and can usually be remedied by time and adequate medical care. In some cases, it is necessary for either the mother or the baby to be hospitalized. If this occurs, there are steps you can take to make sure that you can continue breastfeeding. Even if you have to suspend breastfeeding or use supplemental bottles because of a medical situation, you should eventually be able to resume your normal nursing pattern.

When Your Baby Is Ill

Although breast milk has many protective properties, it cannot totally prevent your baby from getting common illnesses such as colds and the flu. Most breast-fed babies begin to nurse more frequently when they do not feel well. The warmth and closeness of your body and the repetitive motion of suckling will be soothing to your baby when he is ill. Also, increased nursings will provide him with the fluids and nourishment he needs.

In some situations, however, your baby's illness may make him reluctant to nurse. An ear infection or a sore throat may cause nursing to be painful, while a stuffy or runny nose may make breathing difficult. Holding your baby in an upright position during feedings will facilitate drainage in his ears, nose, and throat. If you suspect an ear infection, contact your doctor immediately so that he can provide the necessary treatment. If your baby has a cold, the doctor may instruct you to use an eyedropper to put a few drops of salt water into your baby's nose, or to clear out the mucus with a syringe before nursing.

Whenever your baby has a fever or shows other signs of common illness, he should be seen by a physician. Be sure to remind the doctor that your baby is being breast-fed so that he can prescribe appropriate treatment and coordinate the medication schedule with your nursing schedule. To prevent dehydration, a sick baby should be allowed unrestricted nursings—especially if he has a fever. If your baby is weak or lethargic, he may not cry or otherwise let you know that he wants to nurse. Initiate breastfeeding every few hours, regardless of his apparent lack of interest. Your baby will most likely appreciate every opportunity to nurse.

If your baby comes down with an intestinal virus that causes vomiting or diarrhea, you will probably be able to continue nursing. Many doctors who prescribe "clear fluids only" consider breast milk to be acceptable, as it is easily digested and likely to aid in recovery. Nurse your baby every hour or two for short periods, so that he takes in only small quantities of milk at a time. If his condition does not begin to improve after twenty-four hours, your doctor may recommend that you suspend breastfeeding. Until breastfeeding is resumed, be sure to empty your breasts at regular nursing times in order to maintain your milk supply and prevent plugged ducts.

Although your sick baby will place many demands on your time and energy, take care to satisfy your own needs for sleep and good nutrition. In order to preserve your health and maintain your milk supply, try to nap during the day. As your baby's condition improves, he may begin to sleep for longer periods of time, enabling you to rest and recuperate too. As nursing returns to its previous pattern, you may find that you are producing excess milk because of the increase in feedings that occurred during your child's illness. Express milk for comfort until your supply is again compatible with your baby's needs.

Some ailments in your baby can be transferred to your nipples and cause you discomfort. Be alert to signs that your baby has thrush. Babies sometimes develop this infection after antibiotic treatment, and can pass it on to you, causing sore nipples. See page 101 for more information on thrush and its treatment.

After a fever, your baby may develop fever blisters on his lips or in his mouth. These are painful, and may cause him to refuse to nurse for several days. They can also be passed on to you during the initial stages of infection, ultimately appearing on your nipples. For this reason, if your baby develops fever blisters in his mouth, you may wish to suspend breastfeeding until they have healed.

When You Are Ill

It is almost inevitable that you will suffer from a cold, the flu, or some other common illness while breastfeeding. When you become ill, you may wonder if it is safe for you to nurse your baby. Most of the time, the antibodies you are forming to the disease are passed through your breast milk to your baby. Since viruses are usually spread through the nose and mouth, take care to avoid close facial contact with your baby. Direct mouth contact is especially likely to spread infection. To further protect your baby, remember to use good hand-washing techniques prior to holding him or otherwise caring for him. Check with your baby's doctor about the safety of any medication you are taking, even if it is an over-the-counter drug.

Hospitalization of Mother or Baby

If you are faced with a possible separation from your baby due to his hospitalization, try to work out some type of rooming-in arrangement so that nursing need not be interrupted. In the event that you are unable to stay with him, arrange to be with him for daytime feedings, with the hospital staff giving him a bottle at night. If nursing must be temporarily discontinued, pump to maintain your milk supply, and resume nursing as soon as possible. Spend as much time as you can with your baby, holding, touching, and talking to him to speed his recovery.

If you are to be hospitalized, try to delay any elective procedure until your baby is at least six to eight weeks old, since your milk supply should be well-established by then. Both the reason for your hospitalization and the immediate environment to which your baby will be exposed should be considered. Since many diseases are treated in a hospital, its environment includes many more types of bacteria and viruses than are found in a single home. Therefore, taking your baby into a hospital will increase his exposure to disease-producing organisms. You will need to weigh the risks of taking your baby into the hospital environment against the benefits of continuing to breastfeed. One way to minimize this danger is by arranging for a private room. If your baby cannot stay with you, you may be allowed to have him brought to your room for feedings.

Hospitalization will undoubtedly interrupt your nursing schedule to some degree. Whenever you miss a feeding, try to express or pump your milk in order to maintain your milk supply and avoid engorgement. When your separation ends, you can again adjust your milk supply to suit your baby's needs. The longer the separation, the more time it will take to return to your previous breastfeeding schedule.

When you and your baby are back home, spend as much time together as possible. If your milk supply is low, nurse often. Increased skin contact will be comforting to both of you, and will encourage your baby to nurse. Frequent feedings will provide the stimulation needed for an increase in milk production. If formula supplements are necessary, they should be offered in small quantities, and only after your baby has nursed.

RELACTATION AND ADOPTION

Occasionally, a woman may wish to begin breastfeeding after having previously chosen to formula feed her baby. This is referred to as relactation, since lactation was suppressed either after delivery or after a period of breastfeeding, and was resumed at a later time.

Similarly, some women choose to nurse an adopted baby, and thus must take measures to induce lactation. While total nourishment by breast milk may not be possible in every case of relactation or induced lactation, mother and baby can still enjoy the emotional and physical benefits of breastfeeding.

Such unique endeavors require time, patience, support, and special techniques. Several books, pamphlets, and articles deal with these topics in depth. A lactation consultant or breastfeeding support group should be able to aid you in locating these publications. They will also be able to provide you with practical advice and personal guidance.

While the special situations discussed in this chapter may create complications in the course of your breastfeeding experience, they need not keep you from nursing. By educating yourself about your situation, you will prepare yourself for the necessary adjustments. Naturally, you may have to re-evaluate what you consider to be the ideal nursing relationship. Remember, though, that the ultimate goal of breastfeeding is not the realization of a dream, but the nurturing of a happy, healthy baby.

AT A GLANCE

Nursing in Special Situations

Cesarean Birth

- By using simple aids and techniques, Cesarean mothers can breastfeed successfully.
- Initially, a baby born by Cesarean may be drowsy and have difficulty getting on the breast. Patience is required to initiate breastfeedings.
- A Cesarean mother requires a longer period of recovery, in addition to help at home.

Multiple Births

- You can produce enough milk for more than one baby. Your milk supply will increase in response to the additional amount of suckling.
- Twins can be nursed at the same time or separately. Plan at least one individual feeding a day so that each baby can enjoy a special time alone with you.
- Each twin either can alternate between breasts from feeding to feeding or day to day, or can always nurse on the same breast.
- Triplets can be nursed successfully. Sometimes, a mother can totally breastfeed all three babies. In other cases, one baby will receive a bottle while the other two nurse. At each feeding, a different baby should receive the bottle, so that all babies enjoy the same amount of time at the breast.

The Premature or Ill Newborn

- A baby's ability to begin nursing depends on his birth weight, overall health, sucking reflex, and the medications he is receiving.
- When nursing is delayed at birth, you can build and maintain your milk supply by pumping your breasts regularly.
- The milk of a premie's mother is uniquely suited to meet the needs of her premature baby.
- Your milk can be frozen and saved for your baby. Arrange for the hospital to provide your baby with the expressed milk.
- Spend as much time as possible with your baby.
- When your baby is able to begin nursing, he may tire easily and require lengthy nursing sessions.
- If you have advance notice, pump more often during the week before

your baby comes home. Night pumpings should begin at this time.
- When your baby first comes home, you may need to awaken him for feedings.
- Your baby may find it difficult to switch from the bottle to the breast. A variety of techniques may be used to coax your baby to nurse.

Nursing When Your Baby Is Ill

- Get adequate rest and nutrition when caring for your sick baby.
- When your baby is ill, nurse frequently to supply him with adequate fluids and nourishment.
- If your baby has a stuffy nose or earache, you may have to nurse him in an upright position and contact his doctor for medication.
- Pick up and nurse your feverish baby often. Although he may be too weak to demand feedings, he needs your milk.
- If your baby has an intestinal virus, provide him with short, frequent feedings.

Nursing When You Are Ill

- You can usually continue to nurse when you are ill. In most cases, your body will form antibodies to your illness and pass them on to your baby through your breast milk.
- You can reduce your baby's exposure to your illness by avoiding direct mouth contact and by employing good hand-washing techniques.

Hospitalization of Mother or Baby

- Delay elective procedures until your baby is 6 to 8 weeks old.
- If your are to be hospitalized, weigh the risks of taking your baby into the hospital against the benefits of continuing to breastfeed.
- If your baby is to be hospitalized, request rooming-in or visiting privileges to allow for regular feedings.
- When feedings are missed, pump your milk to maintain your supply.

Adoption and Relactation

- Breastfeeding is possible in cases of relactation and adoption.
- Seek assistance from a lactation consultant who can explain the specific techniques that will enable you to cope with your special situation.

15 Breastfeeding Aids and Techniques

Although breastfeeding is considered to be a natural feeding method, there are several techniques and commercial devices available that, if properly used, can make breastfeeding easier and increase your likelihood of success. Some of these, such as hand techniques, breast shells, pads, lubricants, and nipple shields, can help you deal with special nursing situations. Breast pumps, both hand and electric, can help you to accommodate breastfeeding to your lifestyle. Since you may be interested in some of these devices, it is important to know when they are needed and how they should be used. Sources for the devices available for purchase appear in the Appendices.

HAND TECHNIQUES

Two of the most helpful aids to breastfeeding cost no more than the time it takes to perfect the skills. Breast massage and manual expression are techniques that will be useful to you throughout your months of breastfeeding. At first, you may feel awkward when attempting breast massage or manual expression. With practice, though, you will become proficient at both.

Breast Massage

During pregnancy, breast massage will help you become accustomed to handling your breasts. Once you have begun breastfeeding, this technique will promote relaxation so that your milk will let down more quickly. Breast massage will be useful during the early days of nursing as you set up a breastfeeding routine, and whenever you need to hand express or pump milk from your breasts. During feedings, breast massage will increase milk flow and production. The following steps, which are illustrated in Figure 15.1, will help you to use this technique effectively.

1. Wash your hands with soap and water.
2. Support your breast with one hand.
3. Use the other, flattened hand to exert gentle pressure on your breast, moving from the chest wall toward the nipple.
4. Work toward your nipple from four directions—the top, the inside, and, most important, the bottom and underarm portions of your breast, where most milk ducts are located.
5. Repeat with the other breast.

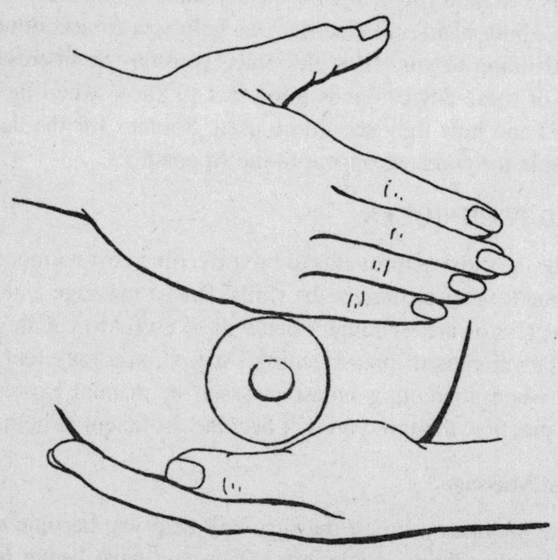

Figure 15.1 Breast Massage

Manual expression

Manual expression will be a useful tool when your breasts are so full that they are difficult to grasp. By expressing a small amount of milk before feedings, you will be able to relieve the fullness and form the breast for your baby. In addition, when used prior to a feeding, manual expression will help to stimulate your letdown reflex before your baby is put to the breast. This will prove useful when your baby is too tired or weak to initiate letdown. It can also be used to alleviate a forceful flow, which is upsetting to some babies.

Many mothers use manual expression on a regular basis as an economical method of providing milk for times they are separated from their baby. Some women have difficulty mastering this skill, and are unable to collect large quantities of milk. Most women, however, are able to express at least enough milk to relieve any uncomfortable breast fullness. It takes time and perseverance to perfect the art of manual expression. Try various methods until you develop a technique that works for you. The most common method of manual expression is depicted in Figure 15.2 and explained on page 216.

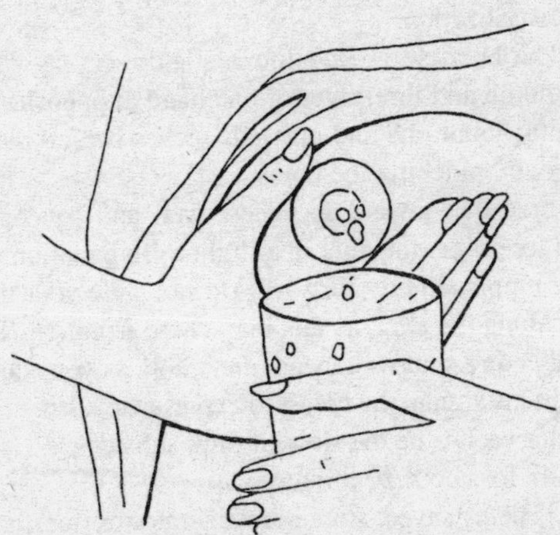

Figure 15.2 Manual Expression of Milk

It is wise to learn how to express your milk manually. Often, occasions arise that make it necessary for you to remove milk from your breasts. Any time you will miss one or more feeding, you will need to express milk. This will serve two purposes. First, it will help to avoid engorgement that could lead to a breast infection. Second, it will help to maintain your milk supply. And, of course, there will be the added benefit of having some of your milk saved for your baby for the next time you are unable to nurse.

By learning the technique of hand expression, you will not have to rely on a breast pump to remove milk from your breasts. Many mothers find this method more convenient and attractive. When preparing for hand expression, you may want to place a towel in front of you to protect your clothing from spraying milk.

Steps in the Manual Expression of Milk

1. Wash your hands with soap and water.
2. If the milk is to be saved for later use, prepare a sterile container to catch and store the milk. (See page 233 for a discussion of sterilization.)
3. Massage your breasts to help stimulate letdown.
4. Place the thumb and forefinger of one hand at opposite sides of the areola, about one and one half inches behind the nipple, as if gently pinching the breast.
5. Press the breast in toward the chest wall and squeeze the thumb and forefinger together in a slight rolling motion while pulling the nipple slightly forward. Do not slide your thumb and finger along the skin, as this may cause irritation. Try to feel the collecting sinuses beneath the areola as you squeeze.
6. Rotate positions around the breast to express the other sinuses.
7. Change sides each time the flow of milk subsides.
8. Express milk for about 20 minutes.
9. If the milk is being saved, store in refrigerator or freezer. (See page 233 for a discussion of milk storage.)

SMALL BREASTFEEDING AIDS

An endless number of devices are marketed for breastfeeding mothers. You may be confused about which devices are really helpful and which should be avoided. Many women enjoy long-term breastfeeding without the use of any devices. However, some situations may arise that require a special breastfeeding aid. Understanding when and how each product should be used will help you to determine its appropriateness in your own nursing management. Because some devices can actually create more problems than they solve, you need to be cautious in your use of breastfeeding aids.

Artificial Breast Lubricants

Most hospitals in the United States continue to give breastfeeding mothers a breast cream, despite the fact that there is no proof that such creams heal sore nipples. If you use a breast lubricant, be sure to select one that will not interfere with breastfeeding.

Artificial breast lubricants should not be applied to a healthy nipple. The Montgomery glands, which appear on the surface of the areola, provide a natural form of lubrication that keeps the skin soft and pliable, provided it is not disturbed. A petroleum-based product will prevent your skin from breathing, while an alcohol-based product will be drying to your skin. Be aware that some wool-based products, such as lanolin, may be a source of potential allergens. Be cautious with the use of Vitamin E also, since safe levels have not yet been determined.

While we do not encourage the use of a lubricant, we do advise that you avoid any product that must be washed off before nursing. The safest lubricant is your own breast milk. Massage a small amount into your breast after you have first allowed the skin to dry well. Avoid applying any artificial lubricant to the end of the nipple where the nipple pores are located. Apply only an amount that can be absorbed into the skin before the next feeding.

Nipple shields

A nipple shield is a rubber nipple that is used to overcome the problems posed by flatness or inversion. This device is placed over the breast at the beginning of a feeding to draw the nipple out, enabling the baby to start nursing. After the nipple is extended, the shield is removed, and the baby nurses directly on the breast. However, a shield should never be used for nipple soreness, as the trapped moisture and increased friction may actually worsen the condition.

A nipple shield can create more problems than it solves! Some shields are made with ridges inside, causing the mother great pain when the baby sucks. Serious complications arise if the shield is left on the nipple too long—especially if it is worn for the entire feeding. The shield does not allow for adequate nipple stimulation, thereby delaying letdown. In the absence of letdown, your baby is prevented from receiving the rich hindmilk that is so vital for his growth. Some brands of shields totally prevent compression of the areola. Poor nipple stimulation inhibits milk production, resulting in a low supply.

Because of these possible consequences, a nipple shield should be used only as a last resort, and only on a temporary basis. Correct use will help you avoid potential problems. Figure 15.3 provides a step-by-step guide to the proper use of a nipple shield.

When using a shield, continue to use other techniques to shape your nipple before and between feedings. Do not allow yourself to become overly dependent on the shield; use it only when absolutely necessary, and then for as short a time as possible. Discontinue its use as soon as you are able. Some babies come to prefer the shield, and refuse to nurse on the breast alone. You can try to wean your baby from the shield by cutting away small sections of the end—a little at a time—before each successive feeding, so that more of your own nipple is taken into the baby's mouth at each nursing.

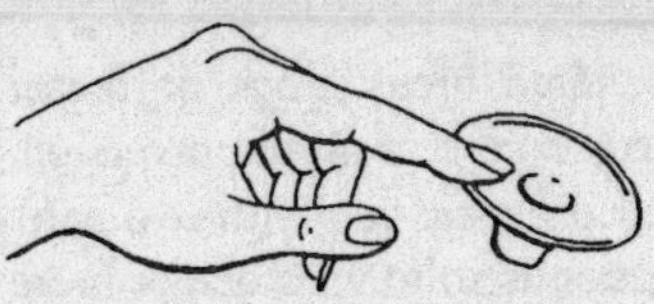

1. Wet the outer edge of the shield with water or breast milk to form a seal.

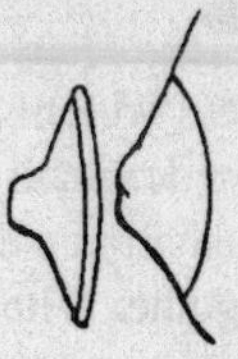

2. Place the shield over your nipple.

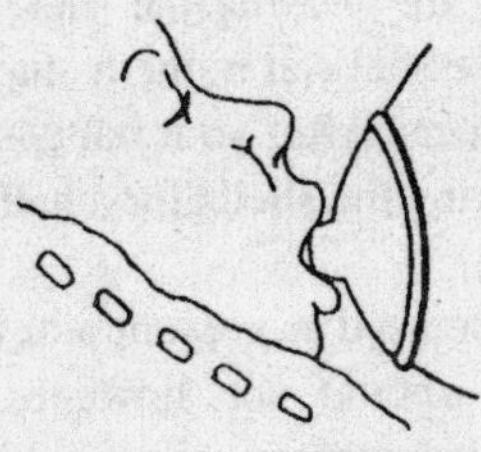

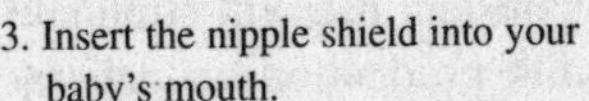

3. Insert the nipple shield into your baby's mouth.

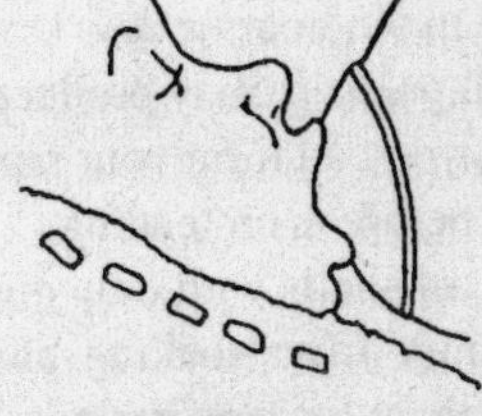

4. Allow your baby to suck on the shield until your own nipple is formed.

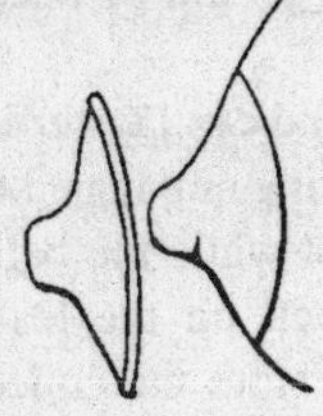

5. Quickly remove your baby from the nipple, then remove the shield.

6. Place your formed nipple into your baby's mouth.

Figure 15.3 Proper Use of Nipple Shield

Breast Shells

Breast shells, which are also called breast cups or breast shields, were originally designed to correct nipple inversion. Each breast shell is a dome-shaped plastic cup with two parts that snap together. The outer section is solid with one or more small air holes; it attaches to the inner section, which has a center opening for the nipple. (See Figure 15.4.)

Placed inside your bra, the shells can be worn for short periods of time (a half an hour to a full hour each day) during the last trimester of pregnancy to draw out an inverted nipple. Gradually increase the time, until you are wearing the shells eight to ten hours a day. Do not wear the shells at night, as the added pressure may produce plugged ducts. After your baby is born, you can form your nipple by wearing the shells for a half hour before each feeding.

Breast shells with only one hole can be used to prevent leaking milk from soaking clothing. You should not, however, wear them for long periods of time for this purpose, nor should you wear them when lying down. Constant use will stimulate the nipple, causing even greater milk production and, therefore, increased leakage. When used for leaking, breast shells should be worn only at those times when leaking would be most embarrassing, and the collected milk should be discarded.

Breast shells that have a single air hole and can be sterilized also provide a means of collecting milk during nursings. Many women experience leaking from one breast while the baby is nursing at the other. If you place the shell on the leaking breast, you will be able to catch and then store the collected milk for relief bottles. To guard against the milk leaking from the shell, be sure to position the breast shell so that the hole is on top. Do not save milk that has been in a breast shell for more than an hour. The following steps should be used when collecting milk in breast shells.

1. Sterilize both the breast shells and the storage container. (See page 233 for a discussion of sterilization.)
2. Have the storage container nearby while you are nursing.
3. As you nurse your baby on one breast, wear the breast shell on the other.
4. Pour your milk into the storage container and place your baby on the second breast.
5. Refrigerate the milk as soon as the feeding is over.

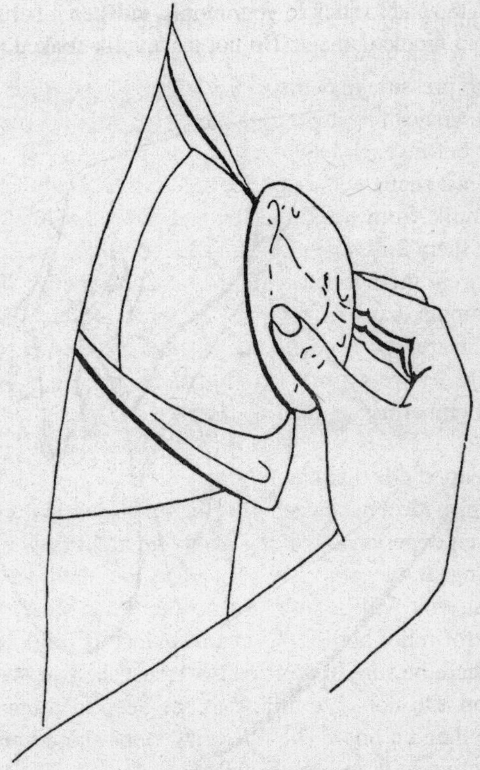

Figure 15.4 Wearing a Breast Shell

6. Freeze the milk if storing it for more than 48 hours.

Breast Pads

Breast pads, which are also called nursing pads, are worn inside the bra to absorb leaking milk. (See Figure 15.5.) The pads recommended for use are those that are made of several layers of cotton. You can fashion your own pads from a portion of a diaper, undershirt, handkerchief, or other cotton fabric. If you prefer disposable pads, avoid those with a plastic layer that can trap moisture against the breast and cause sore nipples. If dried milk causes the pad to stick to your nipple, moisten it before removal to avoid nipple damage. Do not leave milk-soaked pads on for

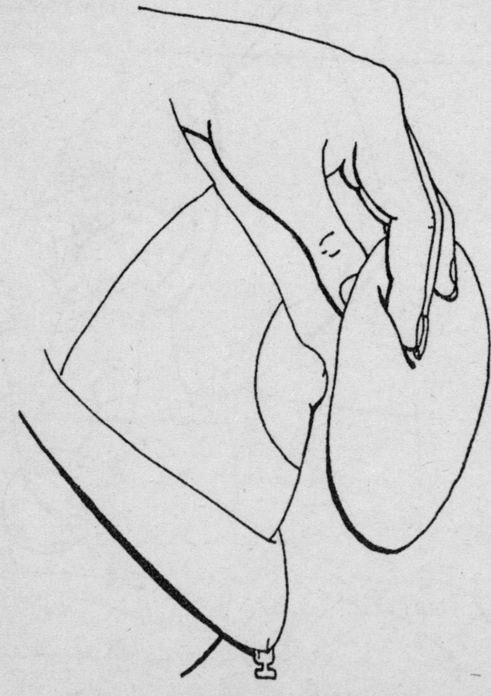

Figure 15.5 Using a Breast Pad

long periods of time, and be sure to air dry your nipples after the pads have been removed.

Nursing Supplementers

Several brands of nursing supplementers have been designed for those breastfeeding women who need extra nipple stimulation and those whose babies need extra nourishment. The supplementer itself is a plastic bag or bottle that either is clipped to the bra or hangs from a cord around the mother's neck. Breast milk or formula is placed in the container and runs through tubing to the baby's mouth. Both the tube and the mother's nipple are placed in the baby's mouth so that he can receive a supplemental feeding while he stimulates the breast to produce milk. (See Figure 15.6.) As the mother's milk supply increases and

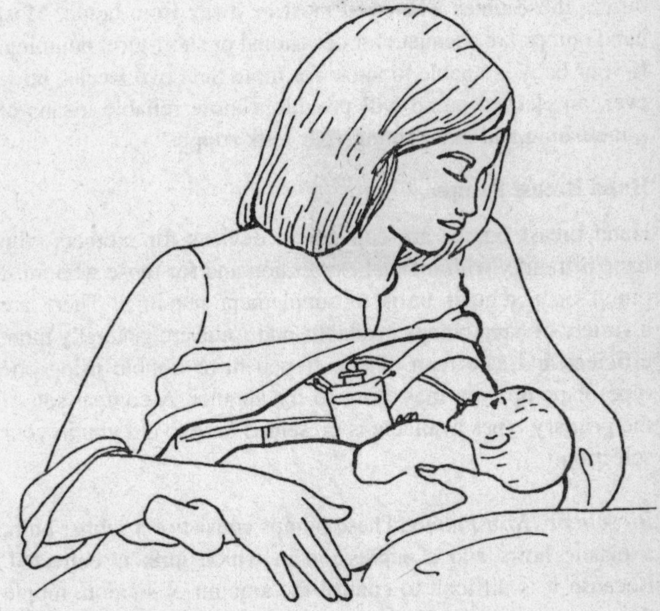

Figure 15.6 Using a Nursing Supplementer

the baby's suckling improves, he takes less and less supplement. Eventually, the nursing supplementer is removed and the baby receives nourishment from the breast alone.

This device has been used for adopted babies, premature babies, and babies with a weak sucking reflex. It has also been used to coax the baby back to the breast after a period of separation, to stimulate milk production when the mother's milk supply is low, and to help induce relactation.

BREAST PUMPS

Breast pumps are available in a remarkable variety of styles. Most breastfeeding women today want a breast pump so that they can provide their babies with relief bottles. Even if you do not anticipate regular separations from your baby, you will find it convenient to have a supply of your own milk on hand for use during those times when you must be away from home. Most hand pumps are adequate for occasional or short-term pumping. If your baby is unable to nurse for more than two weeks, however, an electric pump will provide a more reliable means of establishing and maintaining your milk supply.

Hand Breast Pumps

Hand breast pumps are convenient devices for mothers who have difficulty with manual expression and for those who must pump on a regular basis to supplement nursings. There are a variety of hand pumps available, and some are generally more efficient and safe than others. If you have trouble using one type of pump, you may want to try another. A comparison of the primary types available is presented here to aid you in your selection.

Bicycle or Horn Pumps. These pumps consist of a rubber bulb, a plastic horn, and a depression in which milk is collected. Because it is difficult to control the amount of suction, nipple damage may result. For safety, the bulb should be depressed only halfway. Be aware that the bulb cannot be sterilized, and

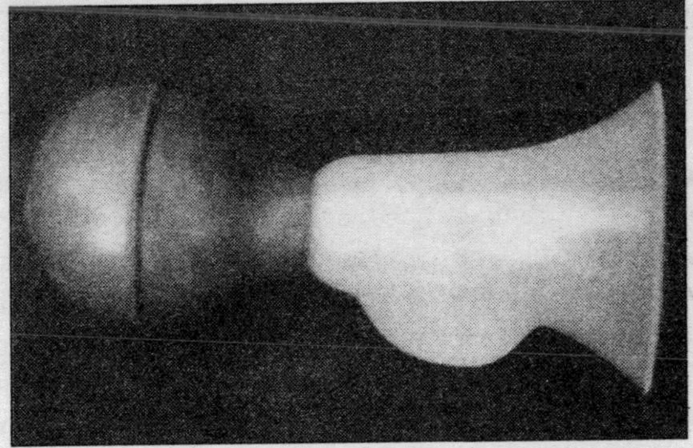

Figure 15.7 Bicycle or Horn Pump

may therefore harbor bacteria that can contaminate the milk. Some common brands are Barum, Davol, and Faultless.

Modified Bulb Pumps

These pumps are composed of a plastic flange and rubber bulb attached to a plastic collecting bottle. They are designed for sav-

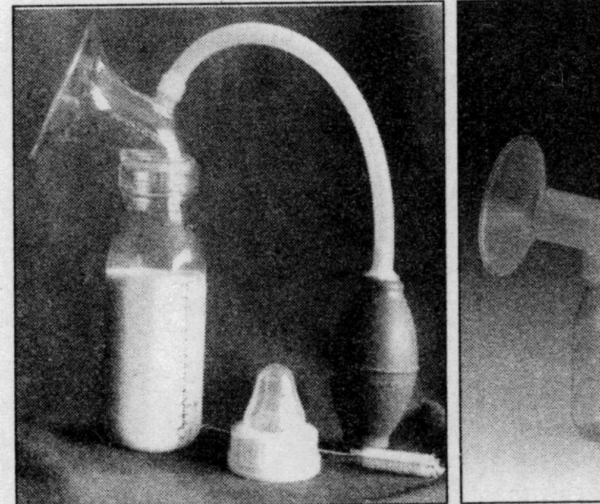

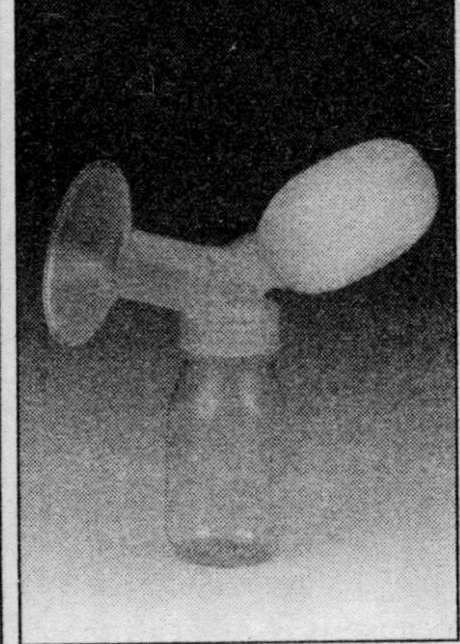

Figure 15.8 Modified Bulb Pump

ing milk, and convert easily to a feeding bottle. Safety may be a concern, however, as the bulb cannot undergo sterilization, and may therefore harbor bacteria that can contaminate the expressed milk. Mothers have reported varying degrees of success in the use of this pump. Popular brands include Evenflo and Le Pump.

Cylindrical Pumps. These pumps consist of two cylindrical tubes that fit inside each other. A vacuum is created when the outer tube is pulled away from the breast. It is easy to control the amount of suction, and users report great success. The pump converts into a handy feeding bottle, and all parts can be sterilized. Brand names include Comfort Plus Kaneson, Crystal, Egnell, Happy Family, Mary Jane, Medela, and White River.

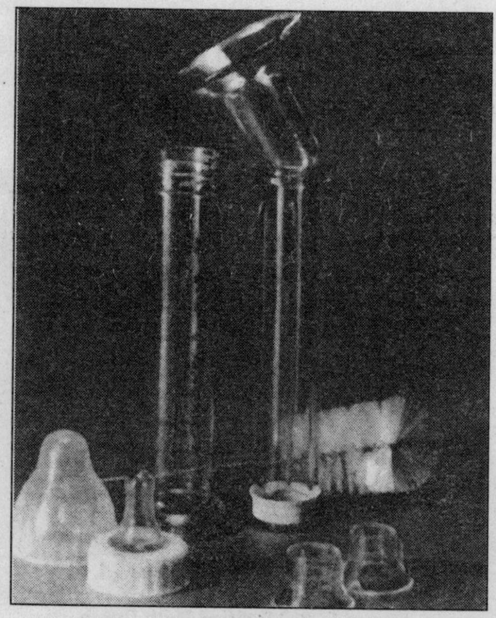

Figure 15.9 Cylindrical Pump

Trigger Pumps. This pump has a glass flange attached to a collection jar. A tube leads from the jar to a trigger, which is squeezed to create a vacuum. A vacuum-relief switch controls the release of suction. Although many mothers have found this to be an adequate means of collecting breast milk, some report difficulty in squeezing the trigger many times in succession and in reaching the suction release mechanism. In addition, the glass collection bottle presents the possibility of breakage. This pump is sold under the name Loyd-B.

Battery-Operated Pumps

One of the newest on the market, this portable pump is powered by two AA batteries. The motor is attached to a plastic feeding bottle and flange. It has an on/off switch, a button for releasing suction, and a knob to control the amount of suction. This pump has the advantage of requiring only one hand for operation. Brands include Egnell Lact-b, Gentle Expressions, Mag Mag, and Natural Choice.

Milk Collection With a Hand Pump

Allow yourself time to develop a routine that will enable you to

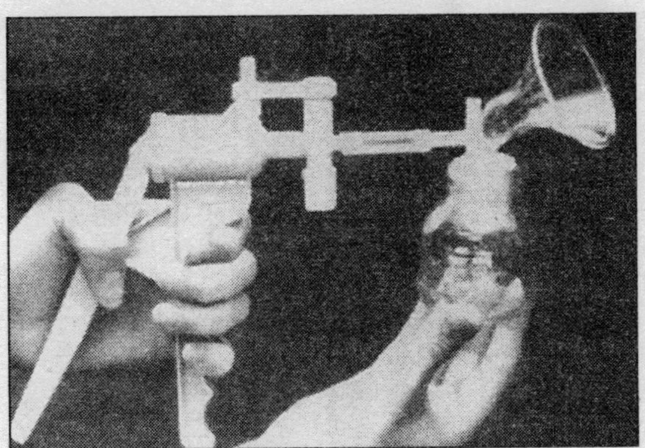

Figure 15.10 Trigger Pump

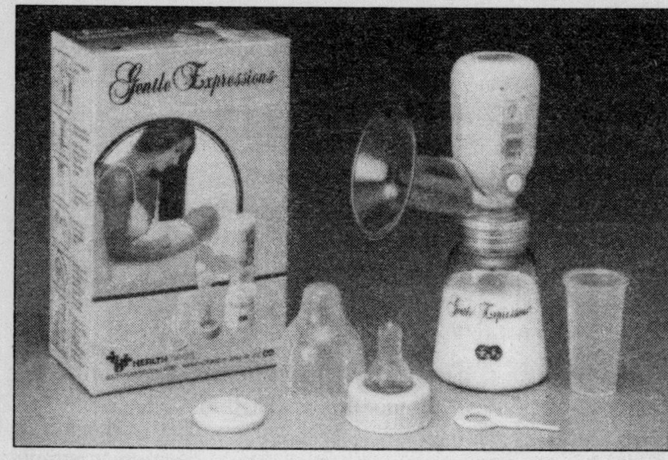

Figure 15.11 Battery-Operated Pump

use the hand pump you have chosen with ease and efficiency. As in the case of hand expression, you will have to determine your own style and technique in order to achieve success. The following steps are suggested for collecting milk with a hand pump.

1. Wash your hands with soap and water.
2. Sterilize equipment. (See page 233 for a discussion of sterilization.)
3. Massage your breasts.
4. Moisten the outer edge of the pump's flange with water or breast milk to ensure good suction.
5. Place the flange on the breast, and begin pumping.
6. Change sides each time the flow of milk subsides.
7. Express milk for about 20 minutes when pumping to collect milk for a relief bottle, and up to 30 minutes when pumping because of a missed feeding.

Electric Breast Pumps

The use of an electric pump is suggested when mother and baby will be separated for two weeks or longer. It provides better nipple stimulation than a hand pump, and is more efficient in emptying the breasts and maintaining milk production. There are two major types of large electric breast pumps available in a variety of brand names, and, despite their size, both types are portable. The automatic type has been found to be more effective than the semi-automatic. Because of the high cost of these devices, mothers usually obtain them on a rental basis. They are also available in most hospitals and clinics.

Recently, a new personal-sized electric pump became available. This device combines the efficient operation of an electric pump with low cost and convenience.

Automatic Suction Pumps. An automatic suction pump has an electric motor and self-pumping action. The mother simply places the flange over her nipple; the pump does all the work. Both the AXi-Care and Egnell pumps are designed for use with a collection packet that includes a collection jar, two sizes of flanges, an overflow bottle, and tubing. Medela sells a combination hand pump/collection device that can be used either with the electric pump or as a separate hand pump. These three brands of electric pumps can be purchased from the manufacturer or rented through pharmacies and private rental stations.

Semi-Automatic Suction Pumps. Semi-automatic pumps were originally adapted from aspirator machines before specially designed breast pumps were available. Suction is created and controlled manually by the mother. The thumb is placed over the valve to create a vacuum, and then released to break suction. The Gomco and Sorenson pumps, which do not include collection equipment, can be found in hospitals, hospital supply stores, and some pharmacies. The White River pump, which comes with collection equipment and carrying case, may be purchased or rented through local distributors. Other semi-automatic pumps include AXi-Care and Precious Care.

Personal-Sized Electric Pumps. Electric pumps are now available in a personal-sized, hand-held model. These pumps combine the efficiency of an electric pump with the low cost and convenience of a hand pump. Suction is controlled by a thumb valve. Brand names include AXi-Care Mini Breast Pump and Precious Care.

Milk Collection With an Electric Pump

An electric breast pump is more efficient than a hand pump. Nevertheless, in order to maximize the amount of milk you collect, you must first condition your letdown reflex by massaging your breasts and relaxing. In the beginning, you may only get a small amount of milk, especially if you have been separated

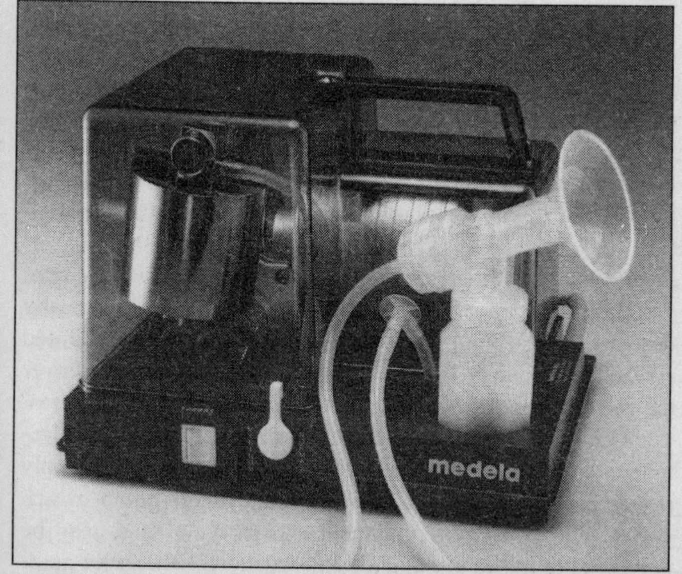

Figure 15.12 Electric Pump

from your baby and have never had the opportunity to nurse him. Once you develop your own style and establish a pumping routine, you will increase the amount of milk you obtain. Follow the instructions recommended by the manufacturer for pump operation. In addition, we suggest these steps for using an electric breast pump:

1. Wash your hands with soap and water.
2. Sterilize equipment. (See page 233 for a discussion of sterilization.) Massage your breasts.
3. Moisten the edge of the flange for better suction.
5. Place the flange over the nipple, and begin pumping.
6. Turn the suction to the lowest level, adjusting the suction for comfort as pumping proceeds.
7. Change sides each time the flow of milk subsides.
8. To ensure an adequate milk supply, pump every 2 or 3 hours for 20- to 30-minute periods. It is not necessary to pump during the night if you are pumping 6 to 8 times per day.

QUESTIONS ABOUT COLLECTING MILK

There are a number of common questions that breastfeeding mothers have about the process of pumping and collecting breast milk. Initially, you may have difficulty achieving letdown when pumping or hand expressing. You may also be concerned about whether pumping will reduce your milk supply, or you may have trouble obtaining the quantity of milk you desire. These are normal concerns. After you have developed your own style and pattern of pumping or expressing, you will discover that you have resolved most of your problems.

What if I don't collect much milk?

If you are worried because you are collecting only a small amount of milk, remember that you cannot remove milk as efficiently as your baby. It takes time and practice to become skilled at pumping and expressing. If you have trouble, rest and try again later. To avoid frustration, spend no more than forty-five minutes at each pumping session. The milk you obtain through pumping is not a true measure of milk production, so do not be alarmed by small amounts.

How can I help my milk to let down?

Just as letdown is the key to successful nursing, so it is the key to obtaining milk when expressing or pumping. You may have to condition this reflex when pumping as you did when nursing. Prepare yourself mentally by relaxing and setting up a routine—find a comfortable chair, get a beverage for yourself, and play soothing music. Pump or express in private when you are rested and unhurried. Use breast massage and slow, deep breathing before beginning to pump. Look at your baby's picture and think of him.

If I pump, will I still have enough milk for my baby?

Do not worry that pumping will reduce the amount of milk your baby gets. Since the quantity of milk is greatest in the morning, you will be able to pump most successfully then. If you pump after a feeding, you will not appreciably reduce the amount of milk your baby gets at the next feeding. If you pump on a regular basis, you may actually increase your supply because of the additional breast stimulation.

If you must pump for an extended period of time because your baby is ill or premature, you may notice that your supply decreases in time. This is because the pump is not as efficient as your baby at emptying your breasts and stimulating your nipples. You will be able to re-establish an adequate milk supply once your baby begins nursing.

What if I collect too much milk?

If you collect more milk that your baby needs, you may be able to donate it to a local milk bank that collects milk for ill babies. There is a great demand for breast milk. Each milk bank has its own procedure for handling milk. Check with your local hospitals to see if there is a milk bank near you.

THE PROPER HANDLING OF BREAST MILK

It is important that the breast milk you pump or express for your baby be handled correctly. This includes the proper care and sterilization of storage equipment. Once you have found the method of collecting breast milk that works best for you, you should carefully follow the guidelines for storing, freezing, and thawing your milk. You can then be sure that your baby will receive the benefits of your breast milk, even when nursings are missed.

Selecting and Caring for Storage Equipment

The first step in the collection of breast milk is the selection of an acceptable storage container. Glass bottles, plastic bottles, and plastic nurser bags each have their advantages and disadvantages. Glass is more easily sterilized and contains no preservatives, but is subject to breakage and may be more difficult to store. Also, some beneficial components of the milk adhere to the glass and are not passed on to the baby. Plastic bottles are easier to store, but care must be taken during the sterilization process. Pre-sterilized nurser bags are convenient and require the least preparation and space to store, but may split when frozen if they are overfilled. They also may explode if sealed while being heated. Please note that all plastic products that are intended to come in contact with food contain preservatives. If this is a concern, glass containers should be used.

In all cases, the equipment in which the milk is to be collected and stored must be sterile. All parts that come in contact with the milk should be placed in boiling water for five minutes, or run through the complete cycle of a dishwasher at the water temperature recommended by the dishwasher manufacturer. If you plan to pump more than once in a day, you can sterilize the collection equipment the first time, and then wash it thoroughly with soap and water after each use throughout the day. Many women find it convenient to sterilize a day's supply of storage containers at one time, inverting them on a clean towel to keep the inside of the containers dust-free.

Storing and Freezing the Milk

It is wise to store breast milk in quantities that your baby will use at one feeding. Three-to-four-ounce portions are suggested for full-term babies, while premies may need as little as one ounce. Milk can be stored in the refrigerator for up to five days, but should be discarded if not used within that time. If you plan to freeze your refrigerated milk, do so within twenty-four hours. Milk can be kept for six months if frozen at O°F or for two weeks in a freezer that keeps ice cream reasonably firm. Follow these steps when freezing milk:

1. The first milk collected in a container may be placed directly in the freezer, with the date of collection marked clearly on the container.
2. When only small amounts of milk have been obtained, cooled milk can be poured onto frozen milk in layers until the desired amount has been accumulated. Be sure to refrigerate the newly collected milk until it is cool before adding it to the frozen milk. (To cool a 4-ounce amount, refrigerate for 6 hours.)
3. When freezing milk, make sure you leave room in the container for expansion. (Place a little over 3 ounces in a 4-ounce container.)

Thawing Milk for Feedings

To ensure that the quality of your milk is preserved, the method of thawing milk should be given as much attention as the method of sterilization. The technique you choose will depend on how quickly your milk must be prepared for your baby. Once milk has been thawed, it cannot be refrozen, and must be used within twenty-four hours. Any of the following methods may be used to thaw breast milk:

- Remove the milk from the freezer and hold the container under running tap water. Begin with cool water, increasing the temperature as the milk thaws. Total thawing time will be anywhere from 5 to 20 minutes, depending on the type of container and the amount of milk.

- Run cool water over the frozen milk until you see that it is beginning to thaw. Then place the bottle of partially thawed milk into a pan of warm—not hot—water. It will take approximately 30 minutes for thawing to be complete.
- Remove the milk from the freezer and place it in the refrigerator. Thawing will take about 12 hours for a 4-ounce container.
- While the use of a microwave oven seems to be a logical way of thawing breast milk quickly, no studies have been done to test its safety. This means that the possibility of long-term harmful effects due to changes in the milk are not known. Therefore, it is not recommended that microwave ovens be used for heating breast milk. If you do choose to use this method, do not use plastic nurser bags, as they may burst. Place frozen milk in the oven, leaving the tops of the bottles open, and defrost on the lowest power setting for 20 seconds. To distribute the heat evenly, let the milk sit for at least one minute, and shake the bottle vigorously. Test the temperature of the milk before offering it to your baby.

The use of various breastfeeding techniques and aids will make it possible for you to overcome many of the temporary difficulties you may encounter, especially in the early days of nursing. With the proper use of these techniques and aids, and attention to the correct methods for collecting and storing your breast milk, you will find that breastfeeding can easily be adapted to your unique needs and lifestyle.

AT A GLANCE

Breastfeeding Aids and Techniques

Breast Massage

- Breast massage can help you to relax before nursing, encouraging your milk to let down.
- Massage may be used to increase milk flow during nursings.
- Always wash your hands before massaging your breasts.
- Concentrate the massage on the lower and underarm portions of your breasts, where most of the milk ducts are located.

Manual Expression

- It takes time and practice to perfect the technique of manual expression.
- To facilitate milk flow, massage your breasts before manually expressing your milk.
- There is more than one technique for manual expression. Experiment to find the method that works best for you.

Breast Lubricants

- Artificial lubricants have not been proven effective as a remedy for sore nipples.
- Petroleum-based creams, which inhibit the skin's ability to breathe, should be avoided.
- Alcohol-based products will dry the skin and should be avoided.
- Safe levels of Vitamin E have not yet been determined.
- Apply lubricants to air-dried skin only, and avoid the end of the nipple.
- Breast milk is the safest lubricant you can use.

Nipple Shields

- A nipple shield can be used to make the nipple more graspable and to get the baby started nursing.
- If a nipple shield is used incorrectly, it may cause many problems for both mother and baby, including a decreased milk

supply and refusal to nurse directly at the breast.

- A nipple shield should never be worn for an entire feeding.
- Before using a nipple shield, all other methods of treatment should be explored.

Breast Shells

- Breast shells can be used to correct inverted nipples, both prenatally and between feedings.
- Breast shells should not be worn when lying down, since the pressure could cause plugged ducts.
- Some breast shells can be sterilized and used to collect leaking milk during feedings. The milk must be refrigerated immediately.
- An extended use of breast shells can cause excessive leaking.

Breast Pads

- Breast pads are worn to absorb leaking milk.
- Avoid pads that have a plastic liner since they can trap moisture and cause nipple soreness.
- Replace breast pads as they become moist.

Nursing Supplementers

- The nursing supplementer was designed to stimulate milk production and provide extra nourishment for the baby during feedings.
- This device can be used to coax the baby back to the breast when the mother's milk supply is low.
- The nursing supplementer can also be used to induce relactation, to induce lactation after adoption, and to compensate for a weak sucking reflex.

Breast Pumps

- Hand pumps are convenient for supplemental pumping, but an electric pump is more efficient if you must maintain your milk supply over a long period of time.
- Different types and brands vary in their effectiveness; choose your pump carefully.

- The parts of the pump that come into contact with your milk must be sterilized if you plan to save the milk.
- When using a breast pump, the edge of the flange should be placed in contact with your nipple to provide the necessary stimulation.
- To obtain good suction, moisten the pump flange before placing it over the nipple.

Collecting Breast Milk

- When you first attempt to collect milk for supplementing, do not be discouraged by the small amount that is produced.
- Always wash your hands and massage your breasts to initiate letdown before expressing or pumping milk.
- Alternate milk expression between your breasts, changing sides as the flow of milk subsides.
- Collect milk in small quantities that your baby will use at one feeding.

Storing Breast Milk

- A variety of storage containers are available. Choose the type that best suits your needs.
- Collect milk in a sterile container and refrigerate it immediately. Milk can be refrigerated for 48 hours, or stored in the freezer at 0°F for 6 months.
- Collected milk can be layered on top of frozen milk to obtain the amount needed for one feeding. Remember to cool the new milk before adding it to the frozen milk.
- Milk can best be thawed in the refrigerator or under running tap water.
- Milk that is not needed by your baby can be donated to milk banks, where it will be made available to sick babies.

Afterword

Breastfeeding is but one of the many rewarding experiences you will encounter during your child's early months. Every new day with your baby will bring a greater awareness and appreciation of his uniqueness. Enjoy this phase of your family's growth, confident in the knowledge that your commitment to breastfeeding will contribute to your baby's health and development.

This book has provided you with a comprehensive overview of breastfeeding management. We hope that it has helped you to understand the benefits of breastfeeding for both you and your baby. You have learned how to prepare for breastfeeding, how the lactating breast functions, and how correct breastfeeding management will establish and maintain a plentiful milk supply. You also know how to eat well for yourself and your baby, and are aware of those substances that you should avoid in order to preserve the quality of your breast milk. In addition, you are familiar with the day-to-day management of feedings, and know how to handle problems when they arise.

Hopefully, your adjustment to parenthood and breastfeeding will be easier as a result of the information provided in this book. You now can appreciate the special rewards of nursing the older-child, and can prepare for the introduction of solid foods and weaning. You should also be able to cope with special nursing situations and separations, and to know when and how to use breastfeeding aids and special techniques.

Most important, we hope that this book will help you to develop a relationship that is rewarding, and that you will be proud of your contribution to your child's well-being. The closeness shared during nursings is unique—in both its immediate benefits to you and your baby, and its long-term benefits to your child's physical health and emotional development. Enjoy your baby, and treasure this special time together!

Footnotes

CHAPTER 1

1. Ruth A. Lawrence, *Breastfeeding: A Guide for the Medical Profession* (St. Louis: C.V. Mosby Co., 1985), pp. 313, 316.

CHAPT ER 4

1. D.R. Lakdawala and E.M. Widdowson, "Vitamin D in Human Milk," *The Lancet*, Vol. 1 (1977), p. 167.
2. B.L. Specker et al., "Sunshine Exposure and Serum 25-hydroxyvitamin D Concentrations in Exclusively Breast-Fed Infants," *Journal of Pediatrics*, Vol. 107 (1985), pp. 372-376.
3. M.A. Siimes et al., "Exclusive Breast-Feeding for Nine Months: Risk of Iron Deficiency," *Journal of Pediatrics*, Vol. 104 (1984), pp. 196–199.
4. R.R. Arnold et al., "A Bacteriocidal Effect for Human Lactoferrin," *Science*, Vol. 197 (1977), pp. 263–264.
5. J.J. Bullen et al., "Iron-Binding Proteins in Milk and Resistance to *Escherichia coli* Infection in Infants," *British Medical Journal*, Vol. 69 (January 1972), pp. 69-77.
6. American Academy of Pediatrics, *Pediatric Nutrition Handbook* (Elk Grove Village, IL: American Academy of Pediatrics, 1985), p. 42.

CHAPTER 5

1. P.J. Illingworth et al., "Diminution in Energy Expenditure During Lactation," British Medical Journal, Vol. 292 (February 15, 1986), pp. 437–439.
2. N.F. Butte et al., "Effect of Maternal Diet and Body Composition on Lactational Performance," *American Journal of Clinical Nutrition*, Vol. 39 (February 1984), pp. 296-306.

CHAPTER 6

1. M.C. Iffrig, Sr., "Nursing Care

and Success in Breast Feeding," *Nursing Clinics of North America*, Vol. 3 (1968), pp. 347-349

2. P.C. Stutte et al., "Altemate Massage in Breastfeeding: New Benefits from an Old Technique," paper presented at Nursing Research Conference, Arizona State University, Tempe, Arizona, February 1986.
3. Sylvia Slaven and David Harvey, "Unlimited Suckling Time Improves Breastfeeding," *The Lancet*, Vol. 1 (February 14, 1981), pp. 392–393.

CHAPTER 7

1. D.F. Hawkins, *Drugs and Pregnancy* (New York: Churchill Livingstone, 1983), pp. 191-199.
2. Manoel De Carvalho et al., "Frequency of Breast-Feeding and Serum Bilirubin Concentration," *American Journal of Diseases of Children*, Vol. 136 (1982), pp. 737-738.
3. Manoel De Carvalho et al., "Effects of Water Supplementation on Physiological Jaundice in Breastfed Babies," *Archives of Disease in Childhood*, Vol. 56 (July 1981), pp. 568-569.

CHAPTER 8

1. Mark Wenneker, "Breast Lumps: Is Caffeine the Culprit?" *Nutrition Action*, Vol. 7 (August 1980), pp. 3-6; J.P. Minton et al., "Caffeine, Cyclic Nucleotides, and Breast Disease," *Surgery*, Vol. 86 (1979), pp. 105–109; J.P. Minton et al., "Response of Fibrocystic Disease to Caffeine Withdrawal and Correlation of Cyclic Nucleotides with Breast Disease," *American Journal of Obstetrics and Gynecology*, Vol. 135 (1979), pp. 157-158.
2. Editors of *Prevention Magazine, The Prevention Guide to Surgery and Its Alternatives* (Emmaus, PA: Rodale Press, 1980), p. 343.
3. Byrne R. Marshall et al., "Sporadic Puerperal Mastitis: An Infection That Need Not Interrupt Lactation," *Journal of the American Medical Association*, Vol. 233 (September 29, 1975), pp. 1377-1379.
4. A. C. Thomsen et al., "Course and Treatment of Milk Stasis, Noninfectious Inflammation of the Breast and Infectious Mastitis in Nursing Women," *American Journal of Obstetrics and Gynecology*, Vol. 149 (1984), pp. 492-495.

CHAPTER 9

1. I. Jakobsson and T. Lindberg, "Cow's Milk Proteins Cause Infantile Colic in Breast-Fed Infants: A Double-Blind Cross-

over Study," *Pediatrics*, Vol. 71 (1983), pp. 268–271.

CHAPTER 10

1. American Academy of Pediatrics and American College of Obstetrics and Gynecology, *Guidelines for Perinatal Care* (Evanston, IL: American Academy of Pediatrics and American College of Obstetrics and Gynecology, 1983), p. 90.
2. Helmuth Vorherr, *The Breast: Morphology, Physiology, and Lactation* (New York: Academic Press, 1974), pp. 118–122.

CHAPTER 12

1. American Academy of Pediatrics, *Pediatric Nutrition Handbook*, (Elk Grove Village, IL: American Academy of Pediatrics, 1985), p. 42.

CHAPTER 13

1. W.B. Pittard et al., "Bacteriostatic Qualities of Human Milk," *Journal of Pediatrics*, Vol. 107 (1985), pp. 240-243.

CHAPTER 14

1. Ruth A. Lawrence, *Breastfeeding: A Guide for the Medical Profession* (St. Louis: C.V. Mosby Co., 1985), pp. 313, 316.

CHAPTER 15

1. C.M. Marx et al., "Vitamin E Concentrations in Serum of Newborn Infants after Topical Use of Vitamin E by Nursing Mothers," *American Journal of Obstetrics and Gynecology*, Vol. 152 (1985), pp. 668–670.

Appendices

Bibliography

BOOKS

Amencan Academy of Pediatrics. *Pediatric Nutrition Handbook*. Elk Grove Village, IL: American Academy of Pediatrics, 1985.

American Academy of Pediatrics and American College of Obstetrics and Gynecology. *Guidelines for Perinatal Care*. Evanston, IL: American Academy of Pediatrics and American College of Obstetrics and Gynecology, 1983.

Arms, Suzanne. *Immaculate Deception*. New York: Bantam Books, 1984.

Berkow, Robert, ed. *Merck Manual*. 14th ed. Rahway, NJ: Merck, Sharp and Dohme, 1982.

Brammer, Lawrence M. *The Helping Relationship—Process and Skills*. New Jersey: Prentice-Hall, 1973.

Brazelton, T. Berry. *Infants and Mothers: Differences in Development*. New York: Dell Publishing Co., 1983.

Brewer, Gail Sforza, and Janice Presser Greene. *Right from the Start: Know the Truth About Diets and Drugs in Pregnancy*. New York: Random House, 1985.

Brewer, Gail Sforza, and Janice Presser Greene. *Right from the Start: Meeting the Challenges of Mothering Your Unborn and Newborn Baby*. Emmaus, PA: Rodale Press, 1981.

Brewster, D.P. *You Can Breastfeed Your Baby . . . Even in Special Situations*. Emmaus, PA: Rodale Press, 1979.

Donovan, Bonnie. *The Cesarean Birth Experience*. Boston: Beacon Press, 1985.

Dunn, Judy. *Distress and Comfort*. Cambridge, MA: Harvard University Press, 1977.

Eiger, Marvin S., and Sally Wendkos Olds. *The Complete Book of Breastfeeding*. New York: Bantam Books, 1986.

Gesell, Arnold et al. *Infant and Child in the Culture of Today*. New York: Harper and Row Publishers, 1974.

Goldfarb, Johanna, and Edith Tibbetts. *Breastfeeding Handbook: A Practical Reference for Physicians, Nurses, and Other Health Professionals*. Hillside, NJ: Enslow Publishers, 1980.

Gray, Henry. *Gray's Anatomy*. New York: Bounty Books, 1977.

Gresh, Sean. *Becoming a Father*. New York: Butterick Publishing, 1980.

Hawkins, D.F. *Drugs and Pregnancy*. New York: Churchill Livingstone, 1983.

Jelliffe, Derrick B., and E.F. Patrice Jelliffe. *Human Milk in the Modern World*. New York: Oxford University Press, 1978.

Johnson, G.T., and S.E. Goldfinger. *The Harvard Medical School Health Letter Book*. Cambridge, MA: Harvard University Press, 1981.

Kippley, John, and Sheila Kippley. *The Art of Natural Family Planning*. New York: The Couple to Couple League, 1984.

Klaus, Marshall H., and John H. Kennel. *Bonding: The Beginnings of Parent-Infant Attachment*. St. Louis: C.V. Mosby Co., 1983.

Lauwers, Judith, Candace Woessner, and CEA of Greater Philadelphia. *Counseling the Nursing Mother: A Reference Handbook for Health Care Providers and Lay Counselors*. Wayne, NJ: Avery Publishing Group, 1983.

Lawrence, Ruth A. *Breastfeeding: A Guide for the Medical Profession*. St. Louis: C.V. Mosby Co., 1985.

Minchin, Maureen. *Breastfeeding Matters*. Victoria, Australia: Dominion Press, 1985.

Minchin, Maureen. *Food For Thought: A Parent's Guide to Food Intolerance*. Victoria, Australia: Dominion Press, 1982.

Montague, Ashley. *Touching: The Human Significance of the Skin*. New York: Harper and Row Publishers, 1972.

Neville, Margaret C., and Marianne R. Neifert, eds. *Lactation:*

Physiology, Nutrition, and Breast-Feeding. New York: Plenum Press, 1983.

Newton, Niles. *Maternal Emotions*. New York: Paul B. Hoeber, Inc., Medical Book Department of Harper & Brothers, 1955.

Price, Anne, and Nancy Bamford. *The Breastteeding Guide for the Working Woman*. New York: Simon and Schuster, 1983.

Pryor, Karen. *Nursing Your Baby*. New York: Pocket Books, Simon and Schuster, 1984.

Raphael, Dana. *The Tender Gift: Breastfeeding*. New York: Schocken Books, 1976.

Riordan, Jan. *A Practical Guide to Breastfeeding*. St. Louis: C.V. Mosby Co., 1983.

Schneider, Vimala. *Infant Massage: A Handbook for Loving Parents*. New York: Bantam Books, 1982.

Shiller, Jack G. *Childhood Illness: A Common Sense Approach*. New York: Stein and Day Publishers, 1974.

Spock, Benjamin, and Michael Rothenberg. *Baby and Child Care*. New York: E.P. Hutton, 1985.

Thevenin, Tine. *The Family Bed: An Age-Old Concept in Child Rearing*. Garden City Park, NY: Avery Publishing Group, 1987.

Vorherr, Helmuth. *The Breast: Morphology, Physiology, and Lactation*. New York: Academic Press, 1974.

White, Burton L. *The First Three Years of Life*. Englewood, NJ: PrenticeHall, 1975.

Worthington-Roberts, Bonnie et al. *Nutrition in Pregnancy and Lactation*. St. Louis: C.V. Mosby Co., 1985.

ARTICLES AND PAMPHLETS

Adams, Simmone O. et al. "Effect of Nutritional Supplementation in Pregnancy." *Journal of the American Dietetic Association*, Vol. 72, February 1978.

American Academy of Pediatrics. "Breastfeeding." *Pediatrics*, Vol. 62, No. 4, October 1978, pp. 591-601.

American Academy of Pediatrics Committee on Nutrition. "Fluoride Supplementation: Revised Dosage Schedule." *Pediatrics*, Vol. 63, No. 1, January 1979, p. 150.

American Academy of Pediatrics Committee on Nutrition. "On the Feeding of Supplemental Foods to Infants." *Pediatrics*, Vol. 65, No. 6, June 1980.

American Academy of Pediatrics Committee on Nutrition. "Vitamin and Mineral Supplement Needs in Normal Children in the United States." *Pediatrics*, Vol. 66, No. 6, December 1980.

Arnold, R.R. "A Bacteriocidal Effect for Human Lactoferrin." *Science*, Vol. 197, 1977.

Atkinson, P.J., and R.R. West. "Loss of Skeletal Calcium in Lactating Women." *Obstetrics and Gynecology*, British Commonwealth, Vol. 77, 1970.

Auerbach, K. G. "Employed Breastfeeding Mothers: Problems They Encounter." *Birth*, Vol. 11, No. 1, Spring 1984.

Auerbach, K.G. "Maternal Employment and Breastfeeding: A Study of 567 Women's Experiences." *American Journal of Diseases in Children*, Vol. 138, 1984, pp. 958-960.

Baggott, James P. "Human Milk: More Than a Nutritious Broth." *Keeping Abreast Journal*, Vol. 3, No. 1, January–March 1978.

Berkenfield, Janet, and Janet Schwartz. "Nutrition Intervention in the Community—The 'WIC' Program." *New England Journal of Medicine*, Vol. 302, No. 5, May 1978.

Berlin, C.M. et al. "Disposition of Dietary Caffeine in Milk, Saliva, and Plasma of Lactating Women." *Pediatrics*, Vol. 73, 1984, pp. 59-63.

Bullen, J.J. et al. "Iron-Binding Proteins in Milk and Resistance to *Escherichia coli* Infection in Infants." *British Medical Journal*, Vol. 69, January 1972.

Butte, N.E et al. "Effect of Matemal Diet and Body Composition on Lactational Performance." *American Journal of Clinical Nutrition*, Vol. 39, 1984.

Canavan, P.A., and C.A. Lewis. "The Cervical Cap: An Alternative Contraceptive." *JOGN Nursing*, Vol. 10, July/ August 1981.

Carey, W.B., and S.C. McDevitt. "Commentary: Measuring Infant Temperament." *Journal of Pediatrics*, Vol. 96, No. 3, March 1980.

Cunningham, Allan S. "Morbidity in Breast-Fed and Artificially Fed Infants II." *Journal of Pediatrics*, Vol. 95, No. 5, November 1979.

De Carvalho, M. et al. "Does the Duration and Frequency of Early Breastfeeding Affect Nipple Pain?" *Birth*, Vol. 11, 1984.

De Carvalho, M. et al. "Effect of Frequent Breast-Feeding on Early Milk Production and Infant Weight Gain." *Pediatrics*, Vol. 72, 1983.

De Carvalho, M. et al. "Effects of Water Supplementation on Physiological Jaundice in Breastfed Babies." *Archives of Disease in Childhood*, Vol. 56, July 1981.

De Carvalho, M. et al. "Fecal Bilirubin Excretion and Serum Bilirubin Concentrations in Breast-Fed and Bottle-Fed Infants." *Journal of Pediatrics*, Vol. 107, 1985.

De Carvalho, M. et al. "Frequency of Breast-Feeding and Serum Bilirubin Concentration." *American Journal of Diseases of Children*, Vol. 136, August 1982.

Drew, J.H. "DIALOGUE: Breastfeeding and Jaundice, Part II, Infant Feeding and Jaundice." *Keeping Abreast Journal*, Vol. 3, January–March 1978.

Duffy, L.C. et al. "The Effects of Infant Feeding on Rotavirus-Induced Gastroenteritis: A Prospective Study." *American Journal of Public Health*, Vol. 76, 1986, pp. 259-263.

Duncan, B. et al. "Iron and the Exclusively Breast-Fed Infant from Birth to Six Months." *Journal of Pediatric Gastroenterology and Nutrition*, Vol. 4, 1985, pp. 421-425.

Dusdieker, L.B. et al. "Effect of Supplemental Fluids on Human Milk Production." *Journal of Pediatrics*, Vol. 106, 1985, pp. 207-211.

Elander, G., and T. Lindberg. "Short Mother-Infant Separation During First Week of Life Influences the Duration of Breastfeeding." *Acta Paediatrica Scandinavica*, Vol. 73, 1984, pp. 237-240.

Elias, M.F. et al. "Sleep/Wake Patterns of Breast-Fed Infants in the First 2 Years of Life." *Pediatrics*, Vol. 77, 1986, pp. 322-329.

"Evaluating Medical Information," *The Harvard Medical School Health Letter*, Vol. 7, No. 1, November 1981.

Fallot, Mary E. et al. "Breast-Feeding Reduces Incidence of Hospital Admissions for Infection in Infants." *Pediatrics*, Vol. 65, No. 6, June 1980.

Foman, S.J. et al. "Recommendations for Feeding Normal Infants." *Pediatrics*, Vol. 63, No. 1, January 1979.

Forman, M.R. et al. "Exclusive Breast-Feeding of Newborns Among Married Women in the United States: The National Natality Surveys of 1969 and 1980." *American Journal of Clinical Nutrition*, Vol. 42, 1985, pp. 864-869.

Friend, B. et al. "The Effect of Processing and Storage on Key Enzymes, B Vitamins, and Lipids of Mature Human Milk. I. Evaluation of Fresh Samples and Effects of Freezing and Frozen Storage." *Pediatric Research*, Vol. 17, 1983, pp. 61–64.

Goldberg, N.M. et al. "Supplementary Water for Breast-Fed Babies in A Hot and Dry Climate—Not Really a Necessity." *Archives of Disease in Childhood*, Vol. 58, No. 1, January 1983.

Goldman, A.S. et al. "Immunologic Components in Human Milk During the Second Year of Lactation." *Acta Paediatrica Scandinavica*, Vol. 72, 1983, pp. 461-462.

Gross, S.J. et al. "Nutritional Composition of Milk Produced by Mothers Delivering Preterm." *Journal of Pediatrics*, Vol. 96, No. 4, April 1980, pp. 641-644.

Gruskay, F.L. "Comparison of Breast, Cow, and Soy Feedings in the Prevention and Onset of Allergic Disease." *Clinical Pediatrics*, Vol. 21, August 1982.

Guthrie, R.A. "DIALOGUE: Breastfeeding and Jaundice, Part II, Breast Milk and Jaundice." *Keeping Abreast Journal*, Vol. 3, January–March 1978.

Haire, Doris et al. "The Pregnant Patient's Bill of Rights/The Pregnant Patient's Responsibilities." *ICEA* reprint.

Heartwell, S., and S. Schlessman. "Risk of Uterine Perforation Among Users of Intrauterine Devices." *Obstetrics and Gynecology*, Vol. 61, 1983, pp. 31-36.

Iffrig, M.C., Sr. "Nursing Care and Success in Breast Feeding." *Nursing Clinics of North America*, Vol. 3, 1968.

Illingworth, P.J. et al. "Diminution in Energy Expenditure During Lactation." *British Medical Journal*, Vol. 292, 1986, pp. 437-441.

Jacobson, J.L. et al. "The Transfer of Polychlorinated Biphenyls (PCBs) and Polybrominated Biphenyls (PBBs) Across the Human Placenta and into Maternal Milk." *American Journal of Public Health*, Vol. 74, 1984, pp. 378-379.

Jakobsson, I. and T. Lindberg. "Cow's Milk Proteins Cause Infantile Colic in Breast-Fed Infants: A Double-Blind Crossover Study." *Pediatrics*, Vol. 71, 1983, pp. 268-271.

Jakobsson, I. et al. "Dietary Bovine beta-lactoglobulin Is Transferred to Human Milk." *Acta Paediatrica Scandinavica*, Vol. 74, 1985, pp. 342-345.

Jatsk, G.V. et al. "Immunological Protection of the Neonatal Gastrointestinal Tract: The Importance of Breast Feeding." *Acta Paediatrica Scandinavica*, Vol. 74, 1985.

Joaquim, M.C. et al. "The Advantages of Human Milk in the Feeding of the Premature Infant." *Journal of Tropical Pediatrics*, Vol. 31, 1985, pp. 43-48.

Kajosaari, M. and U.M. Saarinen. "Prophylaxis of Atopic Disease by Six Months' Total Solid Food Elimination." *Acta Paediatrica Scandinavica*, Vol. 72, 1983, pp. 11-14.

Khin-Maung, U. et al. "Effect on Clinical Outcome of Breast Feeding During Acute Diarrhoea." *British Medical Journal*, Vol. 290, 1985, pp. 587-589.

Koopman, J.S. "Infant Formulas and Gastrointestinal Illness." *American Journal of Public Health*, Vol. 75, 1985.

Kron, R.E. et al. "Newborn Sucking Behavior Affected by Obstetric Sedation." *Pediatrics*, Vol. 37, 1966.

La Leche League International. "Environmental Contaminants in Mother's Milk." La Leche League International, Inc., Information. Sheet No. 78a, January 1977.

Lakdawala, D.R., and E.M. Widdowson. "Vitamin D in Human Milk." *The Lancet*, Vol. 1, No. 8044, January 22, 1977.

Lenfant, Claude, and Barbara M. Liu. "Passive Smokers vs Voluntary Smokers." *New England Journal of Medicine*, Vol. 302, No. 13, March 27, 1980.

Lucas, A. et al. "Pattern of Milk Flow in Breastfed Infants." *The Lancet*, Vol. 2, No. 8133, July 14, 1979.

Luck, W., and H. Nau. "Nicotine and Cotine Concentration in Serum and Milk of Nursing Mothers." *British Journal of Clinical Pharmacology*, Vol. 18, 1984, pp. 9-15.

McDonagh, Antony F. et al. "Blue Light and Bilirubin Excretion." *Science*, Vol. 3, No. 1, Spring 1979.

McKay, Susan, ed. "Physiologic Jaundice of the Newborn." *ICEA Review*, Vol. 3, No. 1, Spring 1979.

McMillan, J.A. et al. "Iron Sufficiency in Breast-Fed Infants and the Availability of Iron from Human Milk." *Pediatrics*, Vol. 58, No. 5, November 1976.

Mandel, H., and M. Berant. "Oral Contraceptives and Breastfeeding: Haematological Effects on the Infant." *Archives of Disease in Childhood*, Vol. 60, 1985, pp. 971-972.

Marks, Meyer B. "Recognizing the Allergic Person." *American Family Physician*, Vol.16, No. 1, July 1977.

Marshall, Byrne R. et al. "Sporadic Puerperal Mastitis: An Infection That Need Not Interrupt Lactation." *Journal of the American Medical Association*, Vol. 233, No. 13, September 29, 1975.

Marx, C.M. et al. "Vitamin E Concentrations in Serum of Newborn Infants After Topical Use of Vitamin E by Nursing Mothers." *American Journal of Obstetrics and Gynecology*, Vol. 152,1985, pp. 668-670.

Matheny, R., and M.F. Picciano."Feeding and Growth Characteristics of Human Milk-Fed Infants." *Journal of the American Dietetic Association*, Vol. 86, 1986, pp. 327–331.

Measel, C.P., and G.C. Anderson. "Nonnutritive Sucking During Tube Feedings: Effect on Clinical Course in Premature Infants." *JOGN Nursing*, Vol. 8, No. 5, September/October 1979.

Meier, P., and E.J. Pugh. "Breastfeeding Behavior of Small Preterm Infants." *The American Journal of Maternal Child Nursing*, Vol. 10, 1985, pp 396-401.

Minton, J.P. et al. "Caffeine, Cyclic Nucleotides, and Breast Disease." *Surgery*, Vol. 86, 1979, pp. 105-109.

Minton, J.P. et al. "Response of Fibrocystic Disease to Caffeine Withdrawal and Correlation of Cyclic Nucleotides with Breast Disease." *American Journal of Obstetrics and Gynecology*, Vol 135, 1979, pp 157–158.

Miranda, R. et al. "Effect of Maternal Nutritional Status on Immunological Substances in Human Colostrum and Milk." *American Journal of Clinical Nutrition*, Vol. 37, 1983, pp 632–640.

Mosher, Marcella R., and Greg Moyer. "PCBs and Breast Milk: Weighing the Risks." *Nutrition Action*, Vol. 7, No. 11, November 1980.

Naeye, Richard L. "Cigarette Smoking and Pregnancy Weight Gain." *The Lancet*, Vol. 1, No. 8171, April 1980.

Nahas, G.G. "Marijuana." *Journal of the American Medical Association*, Vol. 233, No. 1, July 1975.

Nahas, G.G. et al. "Inhibition of Cellular Medicated Immunity in Marijuana Smokers." *Science*, Vol. 193, 1974.

Neifert, M.R. et al. "Lactation Failure Due to Insufficient Glandular Development of the Breast." *Pediatrics*, Vol. 76, 1985, pp. 823–828.

O'Connor, Susan et al. "Reduced Incidence of Parenting Inadequacy Following Rooming-In." *Pediatrics*, Vol. 66, No. 2, August 1980.

Orr, Robin D., and Jeannette J. Simmons. "Nutritional Care in Pregnancy: The Patient's View, Parts I, II and III." *Journal of the American Dietetic Association*, Vol. 75, August 1979.

Pittard, W.B. et al. "Bacteriostatic Qualities of Human Milk." *Journal of Pediatrics*, Vol. 107, 1985, pp. 240-243.

Poland, R.L. "Breast-Milk Jaundice." *Journal of Pediatrics*, Vol. 99, July 1981, pp. 86-88.

Quandt, S.A. "The Effect of Beikost on the Diet of Breast-Fed Infants." *Journal of the American Dietetic Association*, Vol. 84, 1984, pp. 47-51.

Rang, Mary Lu. "Sleep Patterns." *American Baby*, Vol. 43, No. 19, October 1981.

Riordan, Jan, and Betty Ann Countryman. "Basics of Breastfeeding Part V. Self-Care for Continued Breastfeeding." *JOGN Nursing*, Vol. 9, No. 6, December, 1980.

Rogan, Walter J. "The Sources and Routes of Childhood Chemical Exposures." *Journal of Pediatrics*, Vol. 97, No. 5, November 1980.

Rooney, Rita. "Arrangements: How Single Mothers Manage." *Working Mother*, Vol. 5, No. 4, April 1982.

Rosta, J. et al. "Delayed Meconium Passage and Hyperbilirubinemia." *The Lancet*, Vol. 2, November 23, 1968.

Siimes, M.A. et al. "Exclusive Breastfeeding for Nine Months: Risk of Iron Deficiency." *Journal of Pediatrics*, Vol. 104, 1984, pp. 196-199.

Sims, Laura S. "Dietary Status of Lactating Women." *Journal of the American Dietetic Association*, Vol. 73, August 1978.

Slaven, Sylvia, and David Harvey. "Unlimited Suckling Time Improves Breastfeeding." *The Lancet*, Vol. 1, No. 8216, February 14, 1981, pp. 392-393.

Sobel, David. "Don't Let Baby Just Keep Crying, Inattention Now May Cause Real Problems Later." *Philadelphia Bulletin*, November 8, 1981.

Specker, B.L. et al. "Sunshine Exposure and Serum 25-hydroxyvitamin D Concentrations in Exclusively Breast-Fed Infants." *Journal of Pediatrics*, Vol. 107, 1985, pp. 372-376.

Stein, H. et al. "Pooled Pasteurized Breast Milk and Untreated Own Mother's Milk in the Feeding of Very Low Birth Weight Babies: A Randomized Controlled Trial." *Journal of Pediatric Gastroenterology and Nutrition*, Vol. 5, 1986, pp. 242–247.

Sutherland, A., and Auerbach, K.G. "Relactation and Induced Lactation." *Lactation Consultant Series*, Unit 1, Garden City Park, NY: Avery Publishing Group, 1985.

Taylor, P.M. et al. "Early Suckling and Prolonged Breastfeeding." *American Journal of Diseases of Children*, Vol. 140, 1986, pp. 151-154.

Thomas, D.B. "Infant Colic and Drugs in Labour." *The Lancet*, Vol. 1, No. 8217, February 28, 1981.

Thomsen, A.C. et al. "Course and Treatment of Milk Stasis, Noninfectious Inflammation of the Breast, and Infectious Mastitis in Nursing Women." *American Journal of Obstetrics and Gynecology*, Vol. 149, 1984.

Trundle, J.I., and G. C. Skellern. "Gas Chromatographic Determination of Nicotine in Human Breast Milk." *Journal of Clinical Hospital Pharmacology*, Vol. 8, 1983, pp. 289–293.

Wenneker, Mark. "Breast Lumps: Is Caffeine the Culprit?" *Nutrition Action*, Vol. 7, August 1980.

Whichelow, M.J. "Calorie Requirements for Successful Breast-feeding." *Archives of Disease in Childhood*, Vol. 50, 1975.

Whichelow, M.J. "Success and Failure of Breast-Feeding in Relation to Energy Intake." *Proceedings of the Nutrition Society*, Vol. 35, 1976.

Whichelow, M.J., and M. Doddridge. "Lactation in Diabetic Women." *British Medical Journal*, Vol. 287, 1983, pp. 649-650.

Whittlestone, W.G. "The Biological Specificity of Milk." La Leche League International, Information Sheet No. 14, November 1976.

Wickizer, Thomas M., and Lawrence B. Brilliant. "Testing for Polychlorinated Biphenyls in Human Milk." *Pediatrics*, Vol. 68, No. 3, September 1981, pp. 411-415.

Willis, J. "All About Eating For Two." *FDA Consumer*, March 1984.

Sources for Breastfeeding Aids and Devices

Most breastfeeding devices are available in pharmacies and department stores. Or, you may order directly from the company. If you are unable to locate a particular device in your area, the mail order information provided here will enable you to obtain it from the manufacturer or supplier. Whenever a brand name was known, it was noted. Please be aware that sources for these devices change frequently. Some of the products listed below may be discontinued in the future, while new products and sources may become available.

As discussed in the text, discretion should be exercised in the purchase and use of breastfeeding devices. Consult an area lactation consultant if you are uncertain about the advisability of using a particular device. For the name of a lactation consultant near you, you can write the authors at: Breastfeeding Support Consultants, 164 School House Road, Pottstown PA 19464.

BREAST LUBRICANT

Medela, Inc.
6711 Sands Road
P.O. Box 386
Crystal Lake, IL 60014

Lanolin

BREAST PADS

Ameda Egnell, Inc.
765 Industrial Drive
Cary, IL 60013

Bosom Buddies
P.O. Box 6138
Kingston, NY 12401

International Design/ Manufacturing, Inc.
305 Avenue G
Redondo Beach, CA 90277

Comfy-Dri Pads

Medela, Inc.
6711 Sands Road
P.O. Box 386
Crystal Lake, IL 60014

Tamara Dee, Inc.
9057 Greenwod Avenue North
Seattle, WA 98130

Leite Breast Pads

White River
Division of Natural Technologies, Inc.
P.O. Box 1704
Beaverton, OR 97005

Disposable Breast Pads
Washable Breast Pads

BREAST PUMPS

Battery-Operated Breast Pumps

Ameda Egnell, Inc.
765 Industrial Drive
Cary, IL 60013

Lact-b Battery Operated Breast Pump

Graham-Field
400 Rabro Drive East
Hauppauge, NY 11788

Gentle Expressions Breastpump and Feeding System

La Leche League International
9616 Minneapolis Avenue
Franklin Park, IL 60131

Omron Marshall Products, Inc.
600 Barclay Boulevard
Lincolnshire, IL 60069

Mag Mag Battery Operated Breast Pump

Hand-Operated Breast Pumps

Ameda Egnell, Inc.
765 Industrial Drive
Cary, IL 60013

Cylindrical Breast Pump

International Design/ Manufacturing, Inc.
305 Avenue G
Redondo Beach, CA 90277

Cylindrical Breast Pump

Kids Corp International
11500 SW 120th Street
Miami, FL 33176

La Leche League International
9616 Minneapolis Avenue
Franklin Park, IL 60131

Manualelectric Breast Pump

Lopuco
1615 Old Annapolis Road
Woodbine, MD 21797

Loyd-B Trigger Hand Operated Breast Pump

Medela, Inc.
6711 Sands Road
P.O. Box 386
Crystal Lake, IL 60014

Manualelectric Breast Pump

Omron Marshall Products, Inc.
600 Barclay Boulevard
Lincolnshire, IL 60069

Kaneson Cylindrical Breast Pump

White River
Division of Natural Technologies, Inc.
P.O. Box 1704
Beaverton, OR 97005

Electric Breast Pumps

Ameda Egnell, Inc.
765 Industrial Drive
Cary, IL 60013

Bailey Medical Engineering
1820 Donna
Los Osos, CA 93402

Nurture 3

Medela, Inc.
6711 Sands Road
P.O. Box 386
Crystal Lake, IL 60014

White River
Division of Natural Technologies, Inc.
P.O. Box 1704
Beaverton, OR 97005

BREAST SHELLS

Ameda Egnell, Inc.
765 Industrial Drive
Cary, IL 60013

Breastfeeding Support Consultants
164 School House Road
Pottstown, PA 19464

Sunburst Breast Shells

La Leche League International
9616 Minneapolis Avenue
Franklin Park, IL 60131

Breast Shields

Medela, Inc.
6711 Sands Road
P.O. Box 386
Crystal Lake, IL 60014

FREEZING BAGS FOR MILK

Ameda Egnell, Inc.
765 Industrial Drive
Cary, IL 60013

La Leche League International
9616 Minneapolis Avenue
Franklin Park, IL 60131

FUNNELS FOR HAND EXPRESSION

La Leche League International
9616 Minneapolis Avenue
Franklin Park, IL 60131

Medela, Inc.
6711 Sands Road
P.O. Box 386
Crystal Lake, IL 60014

INSULATED CARRIERS

Bosom Buddies
P.O. Box 6138
Kingston, NY 12401

Lac Tote Insulated Carrier

Medela, Inc.
6711 Sands Road
P.O. Box 386
Crystal Lake, IL 60014

NURSING BRA

Bosom Buddies
P.O. Box 6138
Kingston, NY 12401

NURSING GOWNS

Bosom Buddies
P.O. Box 6138
Kingston, NY 12401

Medela, Inc.
6711 Sands Road
P.O. Box 386
Crystal Lake, IL 60014

NURSING PILLOW

Four Dee Products
6014 Lattimer
Houston, TX 77035

Nurse Mate Nursing Pillow

NURSING STOOL

Medela, Inc.
6711 Sands Road
P.O. Box 386
Crystal Lake, IL 60014

NURSING SUPPLEMENTERS

Lact-Aid International, Inc.
P.O. Box 1066
Athens, TN 37303

Lact-Aid Nursing Trainer

La Leche League International
9616 Minneapolis Avenue
Franklin Park, IL 60131

Supplemental Nutrition System

Medela Inc.
6711 Sands Road
P.O. Box 386
Crystal Lake, IL 60014

Supplemental Nutrition System

Resource Groups for the Breastfeeding Mother

BREASTFEEDING SUPPORT GROUPS

Boston Association for Childbirth Education, Nursing Mothers' Council
P.O. Box 29
Newtonville, MA 02160
(617) 244-5120

Promoting breastfeeding as a natural part of the childbearing cycle, BACE is a local group that uses outreach counseling provided by trained counselors to assist women who wish to breastfeed. One-to-one interaction is achieved through telephone contact and at monthly discussions that are tailored to the needs of the women who attend. Supplies and literature are available.

Breastfeeding Support Consultants (BSC)
164 Schoolhouse Road
Pottstown, PA 19464
(215) 326-9343

Breastfeeding Support Consultants provides nationwide training for lactation consultants, breastfeeding support counselors, and childbirth educators, based on outreach counseling and extensive breastfeeding information and research. Supplies and literature for parents and professionals are available.

Childbirth Education Association of Greater Philadelphia, Inc. Nursing Mothers Services
706 Ridge Pike
Lafayette Hill, PA 19444
(215) 828-0131

Viewing breastfeeding as a natural extension of family-centered maternity care and conscious cooperative childbirth, CEA promotes breastfeeding through outreach counseling by trained counselors on a one-to-one basis. Further information and support is provided through monthly discussions tailored to the needs of the local community. Breastfeeding supplies are available.

Health Education Associates, Inc.
8 Jan Sebastian Way (Unit 13)
Sandwich, MA 02563
(508) 888-8044

Health Education Associates provides continuing education programs approved for RNs, RDs, IBCLCs, LPNs, and ICEA childbirth instructors on breastfeeding management for hospital personnel, office nurses, and other health professionals, as well as lay counselors. Pamphlets at different reading levels are available.

International Childbirth Education Association (ICEA)
P.O. Box 20048
Minneapolis, MN 55420
(612) 854-8660

ICEA encourages, supports, and promotes breastfeeding by providing information about resources and making current breastfeeding literature available through the ICEA Bookcenter. In addition, ICEA publishes low-cost, low-reading-level breastfeeding pamphlets. The ICEA Breastfeeding Committee acts as a resource and referral clearinghouse for inquiries.

International Lactation Consultant Association (ILCA)
P.O. Box 4031
University of Virginia Station
Charlottesville, VA 22901

This association for breastfeeding professionals promotes breastfeeding worldwide and can put mothers in touch with the breastfeeding support personnel who work in their communities.

La Leche League International, Inc.
9616 Minneapolis Ave.
Franklin Park, IL 60131
(312) 455-7730

An organization devoted to encouraging women to nurse their babies, LLL provides assistance directly to mothers through local leaders who have had experience with breastfeeding. Phone contact and monthly discussions during which experiences are shared provide the means for leaders to teach mothers the womanly art of breastfeeding. A bimonthly newsletter, literature, pumps, nursing supplementers, and breast shells are available. For a referral to a local leader, a free catalog, or answers to breast-feeding questions, mothers can call 1-800-LA LECHE from 9 AM to 3 PM Central Time, Monday through Friday.

Lactation Associates
254 Conant Road
Weston, MA 02193
(617) 893-3553

Lactation Associates provides health care professionals with training in lactation management. Educational materials, workshops, continuing education programs, and literature for parents and professionals are available.

Canada

Alberta Health
Seventh Street Plaza
10030-107 Street
Edmonton, Alberta T5J 3E4

Health and Welfare Canada
Child and Family Health
Programs, Health Promotion
Directorate
Fourth Floor
Jeanne Mance Building
Tunneys Pasture
Ottawa, Ontario KIA IB4
(613) 957-8342

Infact Canada
10 Trinity Square
Toronto, Ontario M5G IB1
(416) 595-9819

The United Kingdom

Breastfeeding Promotion Group
The National Childbirth Trust
Alexandra House
Oldham Terrace
Acton, London W3 6NH
081-992-8637

La Leche League Great Britain
BM 3424
London WC1N 3XX
(01) 404-5011

A bimonthly newsletter, local discussion groups, and professional publications are available.

Australia

Nursing Mothers of Australia National Headquarters
Glendale Street
Nunawading 3131
Victoria
(03) 877-5011

Nursing Mothers sponsors local discussion groups and provides telephone assistance for breast-feeding women. Literature is available.

PARENT SUPPORT GROUPS

Cleft Palate Foundation
1218 Grandview Avenue
Pittsburgh, PA 15211
(412) 481-1376
(800) 24-CLEFT

This foundation educates and assists the public regarding cleft lip and palate and other craniofacial anomalies. Toll free information, a referral service, brochures, fact sheets, and a quarterly newsletter are available.

Compassionate Friends
P.O. Box 3696
Oak Brook, IL 60522-3696
(708) 990-0010

A self-help organization with over 600 chapters throughout the nation, Compassionate Friends offers support to bereaved parents.

Intensive Caring Unlimited (ICU)
910 Bent Lane
Philadelphia, PA 19118

This parent support organization shares information and resources with parents of premies, parents of high-risk babies, parents who are experiencing a high-risk pregnancy, and bereaved parents. Literature and a bimonthly newsletter are available.

National Down Syndrome Congress
1800 Dempster Street
Park Ridge, IL 60068-1146
(800) 232-NDSC
(312) 823-7550

This organization works at national and local levels to promote the rights and welfare of persons with Down Syndrome; sponsors national and international conventions; and publishes a newsletter.

National Organization of Mothers of Twins Clubs
12404 Princess Jeanne N.E.
Albuquerque, NM 87112-4640
(505) 275-0955

This organization provides information about local groups that meet monthly to discuss twin care and other topics of interest to mothers of multiples.

Index

About the Authors

Candace Woessner, Judith Lauwers, and Barbara Bernard are professional lactation educators and directors with Breastfeeding Support Consultants (BSC), based in Pottstown, Pennsylvania. They have trained hundreds of breastfeeding counselors, and have held several managerial positions in the Childbirth Education Association of Greater Philadelphia.

Presently, they instruct nurses, midwives, dieticians, social workers, consultants, and counselors in breastfeeding management and effective communication skills. Through their courses, consultations, seminars, and workshop presentations, they have established themselves as experts in the field of breastfeeding and lactation. All three are certified through the International Board of Lactation Consultant Examiners (IBLCE) and are members of the International Lactation Consultant Association (ILCA).

Candace Woessner has a Master of Science degree from the University of Michigan and worked for five years as an electrical engineer. She serves as Finance Director for BSC and has a strong interest in nutrition- and lactation-related research. She is also a co-author of *Counseling the Nursing Mother*. Candace served as the president of ILCA during 1986/87, and participated in the writing of the certifying exam for IBLCE in 1987. She and her husband live in Pottstown, Pennsylvania with their two children.

Judith Lauwers holds a Bachelor of Arts degree in English from Michigan State University, with previous pursuits in secondary education, public relations, and volunteer services. Her talent for writing and an interest in communication combine with her position as Program Director for BSC. Judith is a co-author of *Counseling the Nursing Mother*. Her home is in Chalfont, Pennsylvania, along with her husband and two children.

Barbara Bernard is a former special education teacher with a Bachelor of Science degree in Education from Emporia State University. She serves as BSC's Marketing Director, and her special interests lie in testing and statistics. Barbara's training in psychology guides the counseling elements in BSC programming. Barbara, her husband, and their three children reside in Lincoln, Nebraska.